Find It Fast!

Part I: Medical Tests during Pregnancy

Medical tests during pregnancy can be an important part of your prenatal care. Every test provides your doctor with information so he or she can plan the best care for you and your baby. Tests described in this book can help assure you that you both are doing well and anything that might need to be done, can be done.

Many tests are routine tests that every pregnant woman has. Some special tests are done if your doctor thinks he or she could learn more about your health or your baby's health from them.

The first test you will probably have is a *pregnancy test.* This may be done by you at home, or it may be done in a doctor's office. Home pregnancy-test kits are very accurate today.

Once you know you're pregnant, a lot of tests will be done at your first or second visit with your doctor. These tests tell your doctor how healthy you are at this time and whether he or she needs to caution you about certain things to avoid or to watch out for. Some tests are repeated during pregnancy, if necessary.

Every test is important, so participate with your doctor in having them. Keep your appointments for tests, and always check with your doctor's office about test results.

Tests before Pregnancy

Your doctor may conduct some tests *before* you get pregnant, depending on your current medical problems and your family history. These various tests are done to assess your health before pregnancy. If a condition or disease is found that needs to be treated before you get pregnant, it can be done without risk to a developing baby. Some tests you may have include:

- a physical exam, including a pelvic exam—to determine your reproductive health before pregnancy
- Pap smear—an early screening test for cervical cancer
- breast exam
- mammogram, if you are at least 35
- rubella titer—to check for immunity against rubella
- blood type—to determine your blood type (A, B, AB or O)
- Rh-factor—to determine if you are Rh-negative
- a test for hepatitis-B antibodies—to see if you have ever been exposed to hepatitis-B
- screening tests for STDs (sexually transmitted diseases)
- HIV/AIDS test—to determine if you have HIV or AIDS; it is not done routinely (the test cannot be done without your knowledge *and* permission)
- cystic fibrosis screening—to determine whether there is a risk of delivering a child with CF; the

screening test uses a blood sample or a saliva sample

- tests for immunity to various childhood diseases, such as measles and mumps (vaccinations can be done before pregnancy)

Tests for Pregnancy-Related Problems and Situations

- *Hormone levels* may be done before you try to get pregnant. These tests measure the levels of various hormones involved in getting pregnant. Hormones that may be measured include luteinizing hormone (LH), follicle-stimulating hormone (FSH), thyroid-stimulating hormone (TSH) and prolactin level.
- Ask your doctor to test you for *thrombophilia* if you have a family history of the disorder.
- You should also have a test if you have artificial heart valves, a history of rheumatic heart disease with current atrial fibrillation, antithrombin-III deficiency, antiphospholipid syndrome (APS), homozygous factor V Leiden mutation or homozygous prothrombin G20210A mutation, or if you are on chronic anticoagulation medication for recurrent thromboembolism.
- Blood tests that can be performed include the lupus anticoagulant, anticardiolipin antibodies, factor V Leiden mutation, prothrombin G20210A mutation, AT-III antigen activity levels, fasting homocysteine

levels, protein-C antigen activity levels and protein-S antigen activity levels.

- A *pelvic ultrasound* may be done to see if female organs appear normal.
- A *hysterosalpingogram (HSG)* is an X-ray done with dye. Contrast dye is injected through the cervix to examine the Fallopian tubes and lining of the uterus. The cervix, uterus and tubes can be examined to see if female organs are normal.
- Another test, called a *laparoscopy,* may also be done. It is a surgical procedure that can be used to examine the uterus, tubes and ovaries. Laparoscopy is done by placing a small telescope (an endoscope) through a ½-inch incision under the bellybutton (umbilicus). A camera is attached to the laparoscope so pelvic organs can be seen on a screen; they can also be recorded on video and pictures can be taken. A laparoscopy may be done before pregnancy to look for endometriosis, adhesions (scar tissue), cysts on the ovaries or abnormalities of the uterus, such as fibroids.
- *Hysteroscopy* is similar to laparoscopy; a scope is placed through the vagina and cervix to look inside the uterus. A camera is used so pictures can be taken and/or a video can be recorded. The test may be done before pregnancy to look for and to treat fibroids, adhesions or a uterine septum (membrane dividing the uterine cavity).

Tests during the 1st Trimester

Medical tests are important in your prenatal care. These tests can help reassure you that your baby is doing well as it develops, and any necessary actions can be taken. Test results help the doctor determine what treatments may be necessary during this pregnancy or what actions might be taken before another pregnancy is attempted.

The Pregnancy Test

The first challenge of pregnancy may be figuring out if you really are pregnant! Before you buy a home pregnancy test or go to your doctor's office to have a pregnancy test, look for the signs and symptoms of pregnancy, which include:

- missed menstrual period
- nausea, with or without vomiting
- fatigue
- breast changes and breast tenderness
- frequent urination
- new sensitivity or feelings in your pelvic area
- metallic taste in your mouth

If you think you're pregnant, take an at-home pregnancy test. Keep the following in mind.

- Sometimes a woman misses a period because of stress, excessive physical exertion or dieting, and is not pregnant.
- Pregnancy tests have become increasingly sensitive and can show positive results even before you miss a menstrual period.
- Most tests are positive 7 to 10 days after you conceive!
- Most doctors recommend you wait until you miss your period before having a test to save you money and emotional energy.
- Home tests are so accurate now that your doctor may rely on them as an initial screening for pregnancy.
- Your doctor may ask you to do a home pregnancy test when you miss a period to help determine if you are pregnant *before* you go to the office.
- If the test is positive, contact your doctor's office to make your first prenatal appointment.

Routine Tests Done at Every Visit

When you go to prenatal visits, you are weighed, your blood pressure is checked and you may be asked to provide a urine sample. These three simple tests provide a great deal of information.

Pregnancy Tests Can Be Disappointing and Rewarding

Amy hadn't used contraception for a year and wanted very much to get pregnant. She was getting discouraged. Dave and Amy were tired of people telling them to relax and "it will happen." They had done a lot of home pregnancy tests—more than 10 in the last few months.

The next time she was a few days late for her period, Amy decided to be patient. When her period was a week late, she couldn't wait any longer. Without an appointment, Amy went to her doctor's office and asked for a pregnancy test. She provided a urine sample and waited for a few agonizing minutes. She expected another disappointment, another negative test result and more waiting.

She was daydreaming when she heard the nurse saying to her, "Positive, it's positive, Amy, congratulations!" On the way home, she bought one more pregnancy test. She wanted to share her positive test with Dave!

- Gaining too much weight or not gaining enough weight can indicate problems.
- By taking your blood pressure throughout pregnancy, the doctor establishes what is normal for you.
- Changes in blood pressure readings alert the doctor to potential problems.
- High blood pressure can be very significant during pregnancy, especially nearer your due date.

Hearing Baby's Heartbeat Is a Great Experience!

At her second office visit, it was obvious Cindy had been crying. Her eyes were red, and her nose was running. She had a tissue in each hand. She was 12 weeks pregnant.

The nurse took her aside before they went into the examining room and asked her what was wrong. Cindy said she had fallen getting into her car that morning on her way to work. When she got to her office, she realized she was spotting. Miscarriage had been a slight concern for her before, but now she was really upset.

The doctor came in to examine her; it was clear that other than her fall that morning, Cindy's pregnancy was going OK. Using a listening device called a *Doppler,* together they listened to the fast regular *thump, thump, thump* of the baby's heartbeat. Cindy's face was still wet from tears, but her smile came through as she sighed with relief.

At that moment, the door to the exam room opened and Art, her husband, appeared in the doorway, the same worried expression on his face that had been on Cindy's. Realizing that the sound he was hearing was that of his baby and seeing the expression on Cindy's face, he broke into a large smile. They discussed with the doctor signs of miscarriage and things to watch for, but hearing the baby's strong heartbeat made Cindy and Art feel much better.

- A urine sample checks for protein, sugar and bacteria in the urine, which can also indicate problems.

Other tests your doctor may do at office visits include those listed on the next page.

Listen to Baby's Heartbeat at Home!

If you find listening to your growing baby's heartbeat fascinating, and you think you and your partner would like to hear it more often than just at prenatal visits, now you can listen at home! You can rent or purchase a high-quality Doppler to use at home. These portable machines are small, lightweight and easy to use. Ask your doctor about where you can find one in your area. If you can't readily find a machine to rent or to buy, you might want to check the Internet for a reference.

- The doctor listens to the fetal heartbeat with a special listening machine, called a *Doppler* or *doptone.* It magnifies the sound of the baby's heartbeat so it can be heard easily. It is possible to hear the baby's heartbeat around the 12-week visit.
- Measuring the uterus (done in the second half of pregnancy) is another test that helps evaluate fetal growth and well-being. See page 31 for an explanation of how this is done.

Tests at Your 1st or 2nd Prenatal Visit

When you go for your first or second prenatal visit, the doctor will probably order a lot of tests. In addition to a complete physical exam (including a pelvic exam and cervical cultures as needed), Pap smear, breast exam and urinalysis, your doctor will probably have your blood tested. If you have difficulty having your blood drawn or you get lightheaded or faint after blood is taken, you might want to ask your partner to accompany you to these tests. Tests that may be ordered include:

- a complete blood count (CBC) to check iron stores and to check for infections
- a rubella titer for immunity against rubella (German measles)
- blood type to determine your blood type (A, B, AB or O)
- Rh-factor test to determine if you are Rh-negative
- blood-sugar levels to look for diabetes
- urinalysis and urine culture to test for infections and to determine sugar and protein levels
- a test for varicella (chicken pox) to see if you have had this disease in the past
- a test for hepatitis-B antibodies to determine whether you have ever been exposed to hepatitis-B
- a screening test for syphilis (VDRL or ART) to see if you have syphilis; treatment will be started if you are infected (this test is required by law)
- cervical cultures to test for other STDs; when a Pap smear is done, a sample may also be taken to check for chlamydia, gonorrhea or other STDs

- a blood test for thrombophilia
- an HIV/AIDS test to see if you have been infected with the AIDS virus; see page 14 for more information on this important test

Physical and Pelvic Exams

- A physical and a pelvic exam are usually done at the first or second prenatal visit.
- A physical exam is done to check your overall good health.
- A pelvic exam is done to evaluate the size of your uterus, to help the doctor determine how far along in your pregnancy you are and to perform a Pap smear.
- Often at your first prenatal visit, you will have a Pap smear if it has been a year or more since your last test.
- If you have had a normal Pap smear in the last few months, you don't need another one.

Pap Smear

- Pap smears are an early screening test for cervical cancer.
- A Pap smear is done to look for abnormal cells, called *precancerous, dysplastic* or *cancerous* cells, in the cervical area.

- The goal of a Pap smear is to discover problems early so they can be dealt with more easily.
- If you have an abnormal Pap smear, it usually identifies the presence of an infection, a precancerous condition or some other condition.
- Women who deliver vaginally may see a change in abnormal Pap smears; their Pap smear may be normal when repeated after delivery.
- One study showed that 60% of a group of women who had problem Pap smears before birth had normal Pap smears after their babies were born.
- Researchers believe that dilatation of the cervix during labor may slough off the precancerous cells. This is followed by the healing of the cervix as it returns to normal after the birth.
- If your Pap test reveals an infection, it is treated.
- When the Pap smear is abnormal, it can create concern for you and your doctor.
- Testing for human papillomavirus (HPV) may help when the result of a Pap smear is confusing or worrisome. Some types of HPV infection are linked with higher rates of cervical cancer.
- If the HPV test is negative for the type of HPV associated with cervical cancer, it can help reassure you and your doctor that the Pap smear results probably do *not* indicate cervical cancer. You can relax during

Do You Really Need a Pelvic Exam and Pap Smear?

Miranda was very excited about her pregnancy. But the thought of a pelvic exam and Pap smear terrified her. Even though she was 23 and had been married for 2 years, she had been able to avoid the disgusting experience.

Most of her friends hadn't been very encouraging or helpful; they told her horror stories about speculums, stirrups and discomfort. At her first OB visit, Miranda brought her husband Bill along to see if he could help her talk her doctor out of the pelvic exam.

"Won't it make me bleed? Is it really safe for baby? Do I really have to do it?" she pleaded. Her doctor gently explained how important the exam was, especially in pregnancy. She even admitted that she didn't enjoy it when it was time for her pelvic exams either! Miranda reluctantly agreed to have the exam after the doctor told her it could help her baby by allowing the doctor to check the size of Miranda's uterus. This procedure could also help date her pregnancy.

Miranda was very relieved to find the whole exam took less than 5 minutes. It was a little uncomfortable, but it didn't hurt. As she walked out to make her next appointment, the doctor heard Bill remark to Miranda, "That wasn't so bad, was it?" Miranda grimaced but then smiled at him. She'd gotten through it with flying colors.

your pregnancy and wait to have additional tests until after pregnancy.

- The HPV test is performed the same way as a Pap smear.

- If the test reveals a precancerous condition, called *dysplasia*, the next step is usually a colposcopy.
- In a colposcopy, an instrument like a microscope is used to examine your cervix and to look for abnormal areas.
- If any are found, a sample of the tissue is removed, called a *biopsy*. However, a biopsy is usually *not* done while you're pregnant; your doctor may wait until after your baby is born for further testing.
- An abnormal Pap smear during pregnancy is a special situation and must be handled carefully.

Specific Tests during the 1st Trimester

HIV and/or AIDS Test

A test for HIV/AIDS may be done, if you have risk factors that might indicate you could possibly be infected with HIV or have AIDS. There has been much discussion in the medical community about whether all pregnant women should be tested for HIV. Researchers believe the number of babies born with HIV could be reduced if a woman knew her HIV status during pregnancy.

The test can be done with the same blood sample that is used for other prenatal tests; this can help save money. However, the extensive counseling now required *before* the test is given (up to 45 minutes) makes it hard for many doctors to test all pregnant women. Keep in mind the following.

- This test is not done routinely, and it cannot be done without your knowledge *and* permission.
- The ELISA and Western blot tests do *not* reveal whether you have AIDS or if you will get the disease. They can only determine whether you are carrying the virus (HIV).
- If the result of an HIV/AIDS test is negative, you may want a follow-up test in 6 months, if you believe you may have recently been exposed or infected. It can take that long for enough antibodies to form to be detected by the test.

Is an HIV/AIDS Test for You?

Louise was surprised that HIV testing was not a routine part of her prenatal screening tests. She had read a lot about the problems HIV-positive expectant moms could have during pregnancy and breastfeeding. Her lifestyle didn't put her at increased risk for HIV, but she had been injured in an accident a few years ago and had received a blood transfusion while recovering in the hospital.

At her second prenatal visit, she asked about the HIV/AIDS test when the nurse was getting ready to take her blood for the other pregnancy blood tests. She found out they were happy to do the test for her, but she needed to have some counseling before having the test done so she understood the result, positive or negative. They also asked her to sign a consent/release before doing the test.

Antibody Rh-Negative Test

If you are Rh-positive, such as O+, A+, AB+ or B+, you don't need to worry about any of the information in this discussion. At the beginning of pregnancy, blood tests are done to check your blood type, so you should soon know—or be able to find out—if this affects you.

- If tests reveal you are Rh-negative, you'll also be checked for antibodies to Rh-positive blood.
- If you don't have antibodies, you're "unsensitized" (this is good). Most Rh-negative women are unsensitized.
- If you do have antibodies to Rh-positive blood, you are considered "sensitized."
- A woman who is Rh-negative can become sensitized by being exposed to Rh-positive blood.
- Becoming sensitized occurs when Rh-positive blood enters the system of an Rh-negative woman. This can happen during childbirth, with amniocentesis or other invasive procedures, with a blood transfusion, ectopic pregnancy, miscarriage or a traumatic accident during pregnancy, if an Rh-negative woman is carrying an Rh-positive baby.
- The Rh-negative woman reacts to the foreign blood (Rh-positive) by forming antibodies. These antibodies stay in her circulation forever.

- During pregnancy, these antibodies can be a problem because they can cross the placenta. After these antibodies cross the placenta and get into the baby's circulation, they can attack the baby's blood cells. This can make the baby anemic. However, if the baby is also Rh-negative, it's not a problem.
- Also see the discussion of Rh-sensitivity and RhoGAM in the *Medical Procedures during Pregnancy* section, page 91.

Cystic Fibrosis Screening

Cystic fibrosis (CF) is a genetic disorder that causes digestive and breathing problems. Those with the disorder are usually diagnosed early in life. The disorder causes the body to produce sticky mucus that builds up in the lungs, pancreas and other organs. This can lead to respiratory and digestive problems.

With modern technology and new screening tests, today we are able to determine whether there is a risk of delivering a child with CF. Testing for cystic fibrosis is sometimes offered to parents before pregnancy to see if either partner is a carrier of the gene involved. Cystic fibrosis screening is often offered to couples before pregnancy as part of genetic counseling. Testing is a personal decision that you and your partner must make based on the information provided to you by your healthcare team.

- The screening test uses a sample of your blood or saliva.
- Screening is recommended for those at higher risk for CF, such as Caucasians, including Ashkenazi Jews. It is the most common birth defect in this group.
- Whites have a 3% chance of carrying the CF gene; Hispanics have a 2% chance, African Americans a 1½% chance and Asians about a 1% chance.
- One changed copy of a CF gene means that a person is a carrier for cystic fibrosis—a carrier does *not* have CF.
- For a baby to have CF, *both* parents' genes must be altered (each must be a carrier). If only one parent's genes are affected, the baby will *not* have CF.
- Even if both you and your partner do carry the CF gene, your baby will have only a 25% chance of having cystic fibrosis.
- Your chance of carrying the gene for cystic fibrosis increases if someone in your family has CF or is a known carrier. However, you could be a carrier even if no one in your family has CF.
- One test available is called *Cystic Fibrosis (CF) Complete Test;* it can identify more than 1000 mutations of the CF gene. This identification process lets doc-

tors more accurately identify carriers, which can lead to prenatal counseling and diagnosis.

- There are some CF gene mutations the current test cannot detect. This means you could be told you do not carry the gene, when in fact you do carry it. The test cannot detect all CF mutations because researchers do not know all of them at this time. However, unknown CF gene mutations are rare.
- A developing baby can be tested for cystic fibrosis during pregnancy with chorionic villus sampling (see page 25) around the 11th week of pregnancy.
- Amniocentesis (see page 44) may also be used to test the fetus.
- If you believe cystic fibrosis is a serious disorder or if you have a family history of the disease, talk to your physician about this test.

Alpha-Fetoprotein Test (AFP)

The *alpha-fetoprotein (AFP) test* is a blood test done on the mother-to-be to help the doctor predict problems in the baby, such as neural-tube defects, severe kidney or liver disease, esophageal or intestinal blockage, urinary obstruction, fragility of baby's bones and Down syndrome. An AFP test is not performed on all pregnant women, but it is required in some states. If the test is not offered to you, discuss it with your doctor at one of your first prenatal visits.

- Alpha-fetoprotein is produced in the baby's liver, and it passes into the mother-to-be's bloodstream in small quantities, where it can be measured.
- The AFP test is usually performed between 16 and 20 weeks of pregnancy.
- Test results must be correlated with the mother's age and weight, and the gestational age of the fetus.
- If the AFP test detects a possible problem, more-definitive testing is usually ordered.
- AFP detects only about 25% of the cases of Down syndrome; if Down syndrome is indicated by AFP, additional diagnostic tests are usually recommended.
- An important use of the test is to help a woman decide whether to have amniocentesis. If an AFP test is abnormal, one of the next tests that may be done is amniocentesis.
- One problem with AFP testing is a very high number of false-positive results. This means the results say there is a problem when there isn't one.
- If 1,000 women have an AFP test, 40 test results come back "abnormal." Of those 40, only one or two women actually have a problem.
- If you have an AFP test and the result is abnormal, don't panic! You will probably have another AFP

test, and an ultrasound may also be performed. Results from these additional tests should give a clearer answer.

- Be sure you understand what "false-positive" and "false-negative" test results mean. Ask the doctor to explain what each result can mean to you.

Tests Can Help You Make Decisions

Mary and Bob wanted to be "informed future parents," but this AFP test was confusing. It was their choice to have the test; the doctor said it wasn't required during pregnancy. He explained that the test was useful in identifying some problems and those pregnancies at increased risk for Down syndrome and neural-tube defects, such as spina bifida.

The doctor told them one of the problems with an AFP test was *false-positive test results,* which was also confusing to Mary and Bob. He explained that a false-positive result meant the test result was positive, indicating a problem, when there really *wasn't* a problem and everything was OK. He further explained that with an AFP test, very few couples actually had a problem. He went on to add that two other tests, the triple-screen and quad-screen tests, combined a couple of blood tests with the AFP test and lowered the risk of a false-positive result.

The thoughtful, thorough explanation helped Mary and Bob understand that if their test came back positive, there were other tests that could help determine if there was really a problem with their pregnancy. Mary and Bob decided to go ahead with the test to get as much information as they could for the good health of their baby.

Triple-Screen Test

Tests that go beyond alpha-fetoprotein testing are available now to help determine if a fetus might have Down syndrome and to rule out other problems in the pregnancy. They are often called *multiple-marker screening tests* and include the triple-screen test and the quad-screen test (discussed below).

- The *triple-screen test* helps identify problems during pregnancy using three blood components—alpha-fetoprotein, human chorionic gonadotropin (HCG) and unconjugated estriol, a form of estrogen produced by the placenta.
- Abnormal levels of these three blood chemicals can indicate Down syndrome or neural-tube defects.
- The triple-screen test is considered more accurate than the AFP test alone because there are fewer false-positive results with the triple-screen test.
- Higher levels of HCG in your blood, combined with lower levels of AFP and estriol, may indicate a baby has Down syndrome.
- A false-positive test could result from a wrong due date. For instance, if you believe you are 16 weeks pregnant, but are actually 18 weeks pregnant, your hormone levels will appear to be off. This 2-week difference could make the test results incorrect.

- Another reason for inaccurate test results is if you are carrying more than one baby.
- An ultrasound done between 18 and 20 weeks of pregnancy can often answer questions when a test result is positive.
- If you have a positive test result, and your original due date is correct and you're not carrying more than one baby, your doctor may suggest further testing.

Quad-Screen Test

- The *quad-screen test* is like the triple-screen but adds a fourth measurement—the blood level of inhibin-A, a chemical produced by the ovaries and placenta.
- This fourth measurement raises the sensitivity of the standard triple-screen test in determining if a fetus has Down syndrome. It can also predict neural-tube defects, such as spina bifida.
- Measuring the level of inhibin-A increases the detection rate of Down syndrome and lowers the false-positive rate.
- An ultrasound done between 18 and 20 weeks of pregnancy can often answer questions when a test result is positive.

- If you have a positive test result, and your original due date is correct and you're not carrying more than one baby, your doctor may suggest further testing.

Hypothyroidism

Researchers now suggest that women of reproductive age be tested for thyroid-stimulating hormone (TSH). One study showed that after 16 weeks of pregnancy, women who had higher-than-normal levels of TSH had four times the chance of having a miscarriage than women with normal levels. Discuss this test with your doctor if you have any concerns.

I Can't Get Pregnant!

Lisa was the oldest of three sisters. It seemed that her two younger sisters had no trouble getting pregnant and having babies. She couldn't. While her sisters had given their parents five grandchildren, Lisa had had two miscarriages and had been trying to get pregnant again for over a year.

She found it heartbreaking and frustrating to get pregnant, have a miscarriage and not know why it happened, what she did wrong or what she could do different next time. She looked into genetic testing and other medical tests for herself. Her doctor reassured her she didn't need those tests yet. Lisa was a little tired of hearing she should eat right, exercise and take good

(continued on next page)

(continued from previous page)

care of herself, and things would work out, that the two miscarriages were probably bad luck.

Because she was feeling tired all the time, Lisa decided to have a physical exam. Her doctor checked her thyroid and found she had hypothyroidism. She prescribed thyroid medication for Lisa, which helped her feel less tired.

And the medication had another effect. Lisa got pregnant. Her next pregnancy resulted in healthy twin girls!

Chorionic Villus Sampling (CVS)

Chorionic villus sampling (CVS) is used to detect genetic abnormalities; sampling is done early in pregnancy. The test analyzes chorionic villus cells, which eventually become the placenta. The advantage of CVS is the doctor can diagnose a problem fairly early in pregnancy. The test can be done at 9 to 11 weeks instead of 16 to 18 weeks, as with amniocentesis. Some couples choose CVS so they can make an early decision about whether to continue with a pregnancy.

- Over 95% of women who have chorionic villus sampling learn their baby does *not* have the disorder the test was done for.
- To do this test, an instrument is placed through the cervix or through the abdomen using ultrasound guidance to remove a small piece of tissue from the placenta.

- Tissue is then tested for abnormalities that could lead to, or indicate, problems.
- The procedure carries a small risk of miscarriage, so it should be performed only by someone who has experience doing the test.
- The test is usually done in a hospital setting, by a physician skilled in doing the procedure.
- You will probably want your partner or someone else to accompany you to the test to offer moral support and to drive you home when you are finished.

Genetic Tests

There are more than 13,000 inherited gene disorders that we know about. Each year in the U.S., about 150,000 babies are born with some type of birth defect. Some ethnic groups have a higher incidence of specific genetic defects. In addition, certain medications and chemicals can put a couple at risk. Various screening and diagnostic tests may be done to determine whether a developing baby has certain birth defects. If you and your partner undergo genetic counseling, tests may be ordered for both of you. One of the newer tests is for cystic fibrosis, which is discussed on page 17.

Tests may be recommended if your partner is at least 40 years old or if you have had recurrent miscarriages (usually three or more). Testing may also be recommended if you or your partner has:

- a family history of Down syndrome
- mental retardation
- cystic fibrosis
- spina bifida
- muscular dystrophy
- bleeding disorders
- skeletal or bone problems
- dwarfism
- epilepsy
- congenital heart defects
- blindness
- a family history of inherited deafness (prenatal testing can identify congenital deafness caused by the connexin–26 gene)

You may also be offered testing if you and your partner:

- are related (consanguinity)
- are descended from Ashkenazi Jews (risk of Tay-Sachs disease or Canavan's disease)
- are African American (risk of sickle-cell anemia)

The Quantitative HCG Test

A special type of pregnancy test, called a *quantitative HCG test,* may be done in certain situations. It is a blood test done in the 1st trimester when there is concern about miscarriage or ectopic pregnancy.

- The quantitative HCG test measures the hormone HCG (human chorionic gonadotropin), which your body produces early in pregnancy in rapidly increasing amounts.
- A regular pregnancy test, using urine or blood, is based on the HCG found therein.
- Two or more tests done a few days apart identify the change in the amount of the hormone.
- In a normal pregnancy, the HCG level will double every 2 days. If the HCG level is not increasing in this manner, your doctor may be concerned about the possibility of a miscarriage or an ectopic pregnancy. The quantitative HCG can help diagnose the problem.
- An ultrasound may also be done if the HCG test indicates possible problems.

Tests to Avoid during Your Pregnancy

Imaging Tests

- Avoid X-rays during pregnancy, unless it is an emergency.
- There is no known safe amount of radiation from X-ray tests for a developing fetus.

- The medical need for an X-ray must always be weighed against its risk to the pregnancy.
- This warning also applies to dental X-rays.
- Risk to the fetus appears to be the greatest between 8 and 15 weeks of pregnancy.
- Some physicians believe the only safe amount of radiation exposure for a growing baby is no exposure.
- Computerized tomographic scans, also called *CT scans* or *CAT scans*, are specialized X-rays that also include computer analysis.
- Many researchers believe the radiation received from a CT scan is far lower than that from a regular X-ray. However, it is probably wise to avoid even this amount of exposure, if possible.
- Magnetic resonance imaging, also called *MRI*, is often used today.
- No harmful effects have been reported from its use in pregnancy, but pregnant women are advised to avoid MRI during the 1st trimester of pregnancy. Also see the discussion of the ultra-fast MRI on page 34.
- Do not have any test that involves injecting dye into your body.
- If you are not using reliable contraception or there is any possible chance you could be pregnant, avoid or postpone any test involving X-ray exposure until you determine if you are pregnant.

There Are Some Tests You Shouldn't Have during Pregnancy

Elaine was tired of having cramps and diarrhea. She had taken more antacids than food some days. She was sick and tired of being sick and tired and bloated. She didn't know what was wrong.

A couple of doctors had prescribed different diets, but she'd seen only small improvements that didn't last. She was now seeing a G.I. specialist (gastroenterologist) who had suggested more tests. This week he had scheduled her for a series of X-rays, an upper G.I. and a barium enema. But first the doctor wanted her to take a pregnancy test. Her last period was 3 weeks ago, but it was very light. Today she was a little nauseated, which was yet another new symptom!

She didn't think she was pregnant, but she had stopped her birth control a few months ago because she felt so sick. She really wanted to take the battery of tests and get to the bottom of all of this. Elaine thought the idea of a pregnancy test was ridiculous and a waste of money. However, the results changed her mind!

She was 7 weeks pregnant; the tests Elaine was scheduled for would not have been a good idea during pregnancy. Difficult questions would have been raised, such as, "Did the tests harm the baby?" "Should I worry for the whole pregnancy?" "Should I end the pregnancy?"

It's always best to have a pregnancy test *before* any other tests, if there's a chance you might be pregnant. You'll feel better knowing you didn't have any tests done that you should have avoided during pregnancy.

2nd Trimester Tests You May Have

Measuring the Growth of Your Uterus

As your baby grows larger, you will be checked to see how much your uterus has grown since your last visit. Within limits, changing measurements are a sign of baby's well-being and acceptable growth.

- Your doctor may use a measuring tape, or he or she may use fingers to measure by finger breadth.
- Not every doctor measures the same way, not every woman is the same size, and babies vary in size.
- Measurements differ among women and are often different for a woman from one pregnancy to another.
- So if a pregnant friend asks, "How much did you measure?" don't worry if your measurements are different from hers.
- Some doctors measure from your bellybutton.
- Many measure from the pubic symphysis, the place where the pubic bones meet in the middle-lower part of your abdomen.
- Measurements are made from the bellybutton or pubic symphysis to the top of the uterus.
- The top of the uterus is called the *fundus*. Sometimes doctors call these measurements *fundal height* or *fundal measurement.*

- After 20 weeks of pregnancy, you should grow about ½ inch each week. For example, if you are 8 inches at 20 weeks, at your next visit (4 weeks later), you should measure about 10 inches.
- If you measure 11¼ inches at this point in pregnancy (too big), you may need an ultrasound to see if you're carrying twins or to see if your due date is correct.
- If you only measure 6 inches at this point (too small or no growth), it may be a reason to do further evaluation by ultrasound. Your due date could be wrong, or there might be a concern about intrauterine-growth restriction or some other problem.
- Having the same person measure you on a regular basis can be helpful in following your baby's growth.
- If you see a doctor you don't normally see or if you see a new doctor, you may measure differently. This doesn't mean there's a problem or that someone is measuring incorrectly. It's just that everyone measures a little differently.
- If measurements appear abnormal, it can be a warning sign. If you're concerned about your size and the growth of your pregnancy, discuss it with your doctor.

Measuring Your Tummy at Prenatal Visits

Marv could tell that Sondra was tired and a little hurt by people telling her how big she was. "Are you sure it isn't twins?" "Your due date has to be wrong." "Does the doctor say anything about your size?"

These were just some of the uncaring comments she had endured. Marv didn't know how to help and was actually a little concerned himself, although he had been smart enough not to say anything. He decided to go with Sondra to her next prenatal visit; it was his first visit to her OB/GYN.

When it was their turn, Marv noticed that one of the first things done was Sondra's weight check. Before he could ask, the nurse complimented Sondra on how well she was doing with the nutrition and exercise suggestions she had received.

As they sat in the exam room waiting for the doctor, Marv was restless. Sondra seemed to be at ease. The doctor came in, and introductions were made. When Sondra reclined on the exam table, her doctor took out a tape measure, put it on her tummy, then made a notation in the chart. She explained the reason for weighing and measuring pregnant patients was to keep track of baby's growth. She went on to say that women and babies come in different sizes; there wasn't just one size they all fit into.

The doctor explained to Marv that Sondra had asked about her size during a previous visit and was interested in managing her weight gain. Sondra had been given suggestions and was working hard to follow them. Marv decided he would make an effort to attend more office visits. He also made a mental note to stick up for Sondra the next time anyone made a smart remark about her size.

Glucose-Tolerance Test

The *glucose-tolerance test (GTT)* is done to check for gestational diabetes, which occurs *only* during pregnancy. This test is usually done around 28 weeks of pregnancy.

- If you have this test, you will be asked not to eat any food or drink anything other than water after a certain time the night before.
- The next morning at the lab, you will drink a special sugar solution.
- An hour later, blood is drawn to measure the level of sugar in your blood.
- In some cases, blood is drawn at additional intervals.

Ultra-Fast MRI

- A new *ultra-fast MRI* may be used to provide more information on fetal abnormalities.
- It is useful in identifying conjoined twins (Siamese twins), a diaphragmatic hernia, oligohydramnios (little or no amniotic fluid) and various large tumors.
- This test may be done when results of an ultrasound are abnormal or the ultrasound doesn't provide enough information.
- It is considered safe during pregnancy but is used only in special cases.

- At this time, it is not available everywhere, and it is expensive ($1000 to $1400).

Ultrasound

An *ultrasound exam* can be one of the most exciting, fun tests you'll have during pregnancy! It's an enjoyable way to see your baby and, if you have more than one ultrasound, to watch it grow. It's sometimes also a way to identify your baby's sex (though it's not foolproof in this respect). This test is one your partner will probably enjoy as much as you will. Try to arrange for him to come along when it is scheduled, then you can share it together.

- Most women have at least one ultrasound during their pregnancy. Many doctors routinely perform ultrasound on their pregnant patients, but some doctors perform ultrasounds *only* when there is a problem.
- The terms *ultrasound, sonogram* and *sonography* refer to the same test.
- Ultrasound gives a 2-dimensional picture of a developing baby.
- A device emits sound waves, then picks up echoes of those sound waves as they bounce off the baby. A computer then translates them into a picture. This can be compared to radar used by airplanes or ships

to create a picture of the terrain under a night sky or on the ocean floor.

- In some areas, 3-dimensional ultrasound is available; it is discussed on page 42.
- Although the test is usually done at certain times in pregnancy to determine specific information, it can be done just about any time during pregnancy.
- Ultrasound can be very valuable; it helps check for many details of baby's growth and development and has proved very effective in diagnosing some birth defects.
- Ultrasound may sometimes be combined with other tests. For example, when it is combined with the triple-screen test, the combination of the two tests can better predict Down syndrome or trisomy 18, also referred to as *Edward's syndrome.*
- Ultrasound can help evaluate your pregnancy in many ways, including:
  - ~ determining or confirming a due date
  - ~ finding out how many fetuses there are
  - ~ when there is concern about miscarriage or ectopic pregnancy
  - ~ screening for Down syndrome (see nuchal translucency screening, page 44)
  - ~ checking baby's growth

- ~ checking to see if major physical characteristics of the fetus are normal
- ~ seeing if the baby is in the head-down birth presentation
- ~ when baby is in a breech presentation and external cephalic version (ECV) is tried
- ~ looking at a fetus's brain, spine, face, major organs or limbs
- ~ locating the placenta for use with other tests, such as amniocentesis
- ~ providing information on the condition of the placenta, umbilical cord and the amount of amniotic fluid in the uterus
- ~ when there is concern about intrauterine-growth restriction
- ~ when problems with the placenta occur, such as placenta previa or placental abruption
- ~ after a mother-to-be falls or has an accident, and the doctor wants to check on the baby as part of a biophysical profile to check baby's well-being

Where Ultrasound Is Done

- In some cases, a doctor or technician will do an ultrasound in the office during a visit, if the office has ultrasound equipment.

- You may be sent to a lab or radiology department where the test is performed.
- When the test is completed, if there is a problem the doctor may immediately discuss results with you.
- If everything appears normal, you may discuss results at your next prenatal visit.

How Ultrasound Is Done

- Before the test, you may be asked to drink 32 ounces (1 quart) of water. Your bladder lies in front of your uterus; a full bladder pushes the uterus up and out of the pelvic area so it can be seen more easily. Be sure to ask if you will need to drink a lot of water before your test. It is not necessary with every ultrasound.
- You will lie on a table, and the doctor or technician (it depends on where the test is done) will apply gel to your abdominal area.
- A device called a *transducer* will be passed back and forth across your tummy.
- A picture will be produced on the screen of the ultrasound machine.
- The picture may not make much sense to you at first. It may be very difficult to see details. Ask the technician to help you.
- You may be able to take a printed picture of the ultrasound image with you when you leave.

Ultrasound—The Fun Test

Tracey and Elvin had been looking forward to their ultrasound at 18 weeks. Each was sure they knew the sex of their baby. But they couldn't both be right unless they were having a girl *and* a boy! They were so focused on the sex of the baby and who was right and who was wrong, they lost sight of the other benefits of ultrasound.

That all changed when Tracey started bleeding at 17 weeks. Elvin received a frantic call at work from Tracey; she'd had a gush of blood, then spotting after her morning exercises and was terrified she was having a miscarriage. Elvin agreed to meet Tracey at the doctor's office.

In the waiting room, they held hands and even cried a little. Finally it was their turn to go back to the procedure room, where the ultrasound machine was. When the doctor arrived, lubricant was put on Tracey's tummy and the lights were dimmed. They were silent as the ultrasound began. They stared at the screen. At about the same time, Tracey and Elvin could see the baby's heart flickering rapidly on the screen. A big smile appeared on the doctor's face.

Using the ultrasound test, the baby was inspected carefully and so was the placenta. Measurements were taken, and the amount of fluid surrounding the baby noted. There was no obvious reason for the bleeding; everything looked normal.

Tracey and Elvin were reassured and felt a lot better. Tracey listened carefully to the instructions and warnings she was given. It wasn't until later that evening at home they realized they had forgotten to ask if their baby was a girl or a boy!

- You may also be able to have a video made while the test is being done. Ask whether you should bring a new, unused video with you to your ultrasound test.
- If your test is done after 18 weeks, it *may* be possible to determine the sex of your baby, but don't count on it. It isn't always possible to tell the sex if the baby has its legs crossed or is in a breech presentation.
- Even if the technician or your doctor makes a prediction as to the sex of your baby, keep in mind that a prediction of baby's sex by ultrasound is *not* always right.

Ultrasound at the Mall?

Several companies are now offering ultrasounds for your personal enjoyment—these studios can be found in many malls. You can have a 2-dimensional or 3-dimensional ultrasound done, and you may also be able to have a video made of your growing baby.

However, the medical community frowns on this practice. The American College of Obstetricians and Gynecologists (ACOG) advises women not to go to these places. The technicians trained to do the ultrasounds are there to take pictures, not to detect problems. Doctors are concerned that women may not get the prenatal care they need.

If you decide to have an ultrasound at the mall, remember—***a mall ultrasound is not a substitute for a scan from your doctor!***

Some Special Uses of Ultrasound

- Babies with Down syndrome tend to have shorter arms and thicker necks; researchers have developed a method that can be used during a routine ultrasound to help predict a baby's chances of having Down syndrome.
- By measuring the fetal arm and neck, and multiplying it by the mother-to-be's age-related risk of having a Down's baby, the chance of the baby having Down syndrome can be better predicted. For example, a woman of 35 may be told she has a 1 in 270 chance her baby will have Down syndrome. But this test may show that her chance is lower, so she may decide not to have amniocentesis with a risk this low.
- When combined with blood tests (AFP, triple screen, quad screen), ultrasound has been shown to detect Down syndrome in older women (over 35) with a 97.6% accuracy!

Transvaginal Sonography

- Another type of ultrasound is called *vaginal probe ultrasound* or *transvaginal sonography.*
- It can be very helpful in evaluating problems early in pregnancy, such as a possible miscarriage or ectopic

pregnancy, and sometimes gives better information earlier in pregnancy than an abdominal ultrasound.

- For this type of ultrasound, a probe is placed just inside the opening of the vagina.
- The probe does not touch the cervix and will not cause bleeding or miscarriage.
- An advantage of this ultrasound is that you don't need to drink a lot of water or have a full bladder.

3-Dimensional Ultrasound

- In some areas, 3-dimensional ultrasound is being used; however, it is not available everywhere.
- At this time, it is most often used when there is suspicion of abnormalities and the doctor wants to take a closer look.
- A 3-dimensional ultrasound provides clear, detailed pictures of the fetus in the womb. These pictures are so clear that the image almost looks like a picture.
- For you, the test is almost the same as a regular ultrasound. The difference is that computer software "translates" the picture into a 3-D image.
- Doctors have found many uses for 3-D ultrasound, including:
  - ~ improving the measurement of the volume of amniotic fluid
  - ~ showing better pictures of the skull

~ helping to evaluate the baby's spine
~ revealing subtle differences with cleft lip and cleft palate problems involving the face, lips, tooth buds, chin, ears, nose and eyes
~ uncovering defects in the abdominal wall, such as herniated loops of the large and small intestines
~ allowing for better evaluation of the placenta, which can be very helpful if you're carrying more than one baby
~ helping the doctor see some abnormalities of the umbilical cord, such as a two-vessel cord
~ helping to rule out other birth defects

The Cost of Ultrasound

You'll want to ask about cost and coverage *before* you have your ultrasound.

- The cost of an ultrasound varies. An average cost is about $150 but can range from $100 to $300 or more.
- With some insurance plans, ultrasound is an "extra" and not covered under the normal fee for prenatal care.
- Some insurance plans may require preapproval for the test.
- Some plans require that the ultrasound be performed at a specific location or by a specific person.

Nuchal Translucency Screening

- With *nuchal translucency screening,* a detailed ultrasound allows the doctor to measure the space behind baby's neck. When combined with the blood tests, the result of these *two* tests can be used to predict a woman's risk of having a baby with Down syndrome.
- An advantage of nuchal translucency screening is that it can be done at 10 to 14 weeks, so a couple may make earlier decisions regarding the pregnancy, if they choose to do so.
- One study showed that doing this test in women with a higher risk of having a baby with Down syndrome increased the rate of detection of Down syndrome from 60 to 80%.
- When this test is done between 10 and 16 weeks of pregnancy, it accurately detects Down syndrome more than 95% of the time.

Amniocentesis

- Amniocentesis is a test that removes amniotic fluid from the amniotic sac for testing.
- The test can identify about 40 fetal abnormalities (out of 400). It is often used to screen for chromosomal defects, such as Down syndrome, and some

specific gene defects, including cystic fibrosis and sickle-cell disease.

- Amniocentesis may also be done to see if the baby of a sensitized Rh-negative woman is having problems.
- Toward the end of a pregnancy, the test may be done to determine if fetal lungs are mature.
- Amniocentesis can also determine baby's sex. However, the test is not used just for this purpose, except in cases in which baby's sex could predict a problem, such as hemophilia or certain types of muscular dystrophy that occur more often in males.
- In some instances, amniocentesis is done to check for infections or meconium in amniotic fluid.
- Amniocentesis is usually performed for prenatal evaluation around 16 to 18 weeks of pregnancy, making it more difficult to end a pregnancy (if that is what a couple chooses).
- Some doctors now do the test at around 11 or 12 weeks; however, this early use is considered experimental.
- Over 95% of women who have the test learn their baby does *not* have the disorder the test was done for!

How Amniocentesis Is Done

- You will probably want your partner or someone else to accompany you to the test to offer moral support and to drive you home when you are finished.

Amniocentesis—Is It Right for You?

It didn't seem like a time to be arguing, but Ginger and Brett couldn't agree and they needed to decide soon. At 39, this was Ginger's first pregnancy, and Brett, age 40, was new at this, too.

The doctor wanted to know if they wanted an amniocentesis because of their age. That meant putting a needle through the uterus into the amniotic cavity. Ginger wanted the test done; she wanted the information the doctor told them they would learn from the test. She reasoned that she might not do anything about the information if it was negative (Down syndrome or other problems); she just wanted to know ahead of time and to be prepared.

Brett was afraid of the test. He didn't want the risk of miscarriage associated with the procedure, even though it was considered a routine procedure. This was a premium pregnancy!

In the end, Ginger and Brett were able to make a decision. Their years of infertility had drawn them together as a team. They had learned how to consider the entire situation and to make a decision together.

- The test is usually done in a hospital setting, by a physician skilled in doing the procedure.
- Ultrasound locates a pocket of fluid where the fetus and placenta are not in the way.
- Skin over the mother's abdomen is cleaned and numbed with a local anesthetic.

- A needle is passed through the abdomen into the uterus, and fluid is withdrawn with a syringe.
- About 1 ounce of amniotic fluid is needed to perform tests; if you are carrying twins, fluid is often taken from each sac.
- Cells are extracted from the fluid and grown for a period of 7 to 10 days.
- On rare occasions, cells do not grow, so the procedure must be repeated. However, don't panic. This situation does *not* mean the fetus has a problem.

The Risks of Amniocentesis

- Although risks are relatively small, there is some risk associated with the procedure, including trauma to the fetus, trauma to the placenta or umbilical cord, infection, miscarriage or premature labor.
- Fetal loss from complications related to amniocentesis is estimated to be between 0.3 and 3%.
- Discuss risks with the doctor before you decide whether you will have the test.

Blood Tests You May Have for Specific Problems

- *Familial Mediterranean fever* is found in people of Armenian, Arabic, Turkish and Sephardic Jewish background.

- Prenatal testing helps identify carriers of the recessive gene so diagnosis can be made quickly in a newborn to avoid a potentially fatal medical problem.
- *Tay-Sachs disease* and *Canavan's disease* is most commonly found in people of Ashkenazi Jewish background.
- Screening for these two diseases can be done at the same time to determine if a fetus is affected.
- *Congenital deafness caused by the connexin-26 gene* may occur if a couple has a family history of inherited deafness.
- This test may identify the problem before a baby's birth. With early identification, measures can be taken to manage the problem immediately after baby is born.

Other Tests You May Have

Fetoscopy

Fetoscopy enables a doctor to look through a fetoscope to detect subtle abnormalities and problems in a fetus or the placenta as early as 10 weeks into development. Ultrasound may not provide the same degree of detail.

- Fetoscopy is usually recommended only if a woman has already given birth to a child with a birth defect that cannot be detected by any other test.
- The risk of miscarriage is 3 to 4%.
- The test is performed by making a small incision in the mother's abdomen.
- A scope similar to the one used in laparoscopy is placed through the abdomen and the wall of the uterus. The doctor uses the fetoscope to examine the fetus and placenta.
- The test is usually done in a hospital setting.
- Fetoscopy is a specialized test and should be done only by someone experienced at performing it.
- If your doctor suggests fetoscopy, you and your partner should discuss it with him or her at a prenatal visit.
- You will probably want your partner or someone else to accompany you to the test to offer moral support and to drive you home when you are finished.

Percutaneous Umbilical Blood Sampling (PUBS) or Cordocentesis

- *Percutaneous umbilical blood sampling* (PUBS) is a test done on the fetus while it is still in the womb.

- This test has improved the diagnosis and treatment of Rh-incompatibility, blood disorders and infections.
- It can help prevent life-threatening anemia that can develop if the mother-to-be is sensitized and the fetus has Rh-positive blood. For more information on Rh-sensitivity, see page 91.
- Guided by ultrasound, the physician inserts a fine needle through a woman's abdomen into the uterus, to a vein in the umbilical cord of the fetus.
- A small sample of the baby's blood is removed for analysis.
- If a problem is found, a blood transfusion can be done if it is deemed necessary.
- The advantage of the test is that results are available within a few days.
- The disadvantage is it carries a slightly higher risk of miscarriage than amniocentesis.
- The test is usually done in a hospital setting, by a physician skilled in doing the procedure.
- You will probably want your partner or someone else to accompany you to the test to offer moral support and to drive you home when you are finished.

Fetal Fibronectin (fFN) Test

- *Fetal fibronectin* (fFN) is a protein found in vaginal secretions up to about 20 weeks of pregnancy.

- If a doctor believes you may be going into premature labor, he or she may decide to do the fFN test to see if there is a risk for premature delivery.
- The test is done the same way as a Pap smear is performed.
- A swab of cervical-vaginal secretions is taken from the top of the vagina, behind the cervix. The secretion is then sent to the lab, where it is tested for fFN. Results are available within 24 hours.
- If fFN is present after 22 weeks, it indicates increased risk for preterm delivery.
- If it is absent, the risk is low, and the woman probably won't deliver in the next 2 weeks.
- There is a lower risk of preterm birth when the test result for fFN is negative after 22 weeks and before 35 weeks of pregnancy.
- A negative fetal fibronectin test is useful in ruling out impending preterm labor.

Tests for the Woman Expecting More than One Baby

If you are carrying more than one baby, your pregnancy will be different. Even the number of tests you receive, and when you receive them, will be different. In many cases, screening tests give the first indication a woman is carrying more than one baby.

- Some medical experts recommend that if you are at least 32 years old and your doctor determines you are carrying more than one baby, you should be offered chromosome testing, such as amniocentesis or chorionic villus sampling.
- Research indicates there is a slightly higher chance of abnormalities when a woman is carrying two or more babies.

Fetal Fibronectin Helps Detect Premature Labor

Elaine and Billy knew what a premature delivery meant from personal experience. Their first baby, George, was delivered at 29 weeks. Things turned out OK; to look at George today, you'd never know what they had all gone through. They had experienced days, nights and weeks in the intensive-care nursery. The couple and their little baby had endured many tests, shared concerns with family and friends, survived worry and been faced with thousands of dollars in medical bills.

At 24 weeks into her second pregnancy, Elaine started having contractions during the night. She was fairly certain her water hadn't broken. After a phone call to the doctor, Elaine and Billy

(continued on next page)

(continued from previous page)

arrived at labor and delivery just as the sun came up. Elaine knew she didn't want to be there yet—it was too soon for her baby to be born.

After checking in, Elaine was led into an evaluation room, where she climbed into bed. Her vital signs were taken, and a monitor was placed on her abdomen. Elaine had done this with her first delivery; from the monitors, she recognized the strong fetal heartbeat along the top of the strip. But at the bottom of the strip, she saw bumps that she knew were uterine contractions. Her contractions were between 2 and 8 minutes apart but not regular.

Twenty minutes later, after asking many questions, the labor nurse explained that Elaine's doctor would be coming in soon to do some tests. Besides checking her for ruptured membranes, they would do a fetal fibronectin test. She said a swab would be used to remove some secretions from the top of Elaine's vagina near the cervix, and this would be tested for fibronectin. The nurse explained that fibronectin is present in the secretions of the cervix and vagina in normal pregnancies at term but should not be present this early in pregnancy.

Elaine and Billy were told that a negative result (no fetal fibronectin) would be good, predicting that Elaine was not likely to have a preterm delivery. A positive test result (presence of fetal fibronectin) might indicate premature labor and a preterm birth. A positive test wouldn't mean a premature delivery for sure, but Elaine knew she would rather have the test come back negative.

The explanation they received from the nurse helped them relax, and they noticed on the monitor the contractions were getting farther apart. They were able to chat quietly while they waited for the doctor to arrive.

- An abnormal test result does not necessarily indicate the babies have a problem; it alerts the doctor to perform follow-up tests.
- Often with a multiple pregnancy, blood tests are repeated around week 28 to check for gestational diabetes.
- Blood tests can also reveal if a mother-to-be is anemic, which is more common in women carrying multiples.
- Amniocentesis may be done to check lung maturity in the babies if there is an indication of preterm labor or pre-eclampsia in the mother. Respiratory distress syndrome can be a serious complication for multiples who are delivered too early.
- Some of the other tests discussed previously may also be performed if other problems develop.

3rd Trimester Tests You May Have

Group-B Streptococcus Infection Test

Infection with *group-B streptococcus* (GBS) is fairly common in pregnant women—10 to 30% are colonized (see next page). This infection is different from the streptococcus (strep) infection that causes strep throat.

- It is possible to have GBS in your system and not be sick or have any symptoms.

- When GBS is present but doesn't cause infection, a person is considered *colonized.* If a pregnant woman is colonized, it may not cause her any problem but can cause life-threatening infections for a newborn.
- GBS is often transmitted from person to person by sexual contact. In women, GBS is most often found in the vagina or rectum.
- Women who have risk factors for GBS (see next page) are often treated during labor, even if they haven't been tested before.
- Some doctors test all patients routinely for GBS during pregnancy.
- In testing for GBS, swab samples (cultures) are taken from the expectant woman's vagina, perineum and rectum to check for GBS. A urine test may also be done.
- It may take up to 2 days to get the results of your GBS test.
- If the test is positive, a woman may be treated with antibiotics at that time. Or antibiotics may be given during labor. Appropriate precautions can be taken during labor and delivery.
- If a woman is treated for GBS during pregnancy, she may become positive again before her baby is born.
- The best way to prevent GBS in newborns is to treat the woman with antibiotics during labor.

Group-B Streptococcus (GBS)—You Might not Know You Have It

Andi's pregnancy had been perfect so far. She and Sean had just talked about trying to start their family, and it happened! She hadn't had much morning sickness, weight gain hadn't been a problem, she continued working and her ultrasound had even predicted the sex of the baby to be a boy, making both of them happy.

At 35 weeks, she was at lunch with her friend, Nettie; Andi couldn't believe what she was hearing. Nettie's pregnancy had gone well until 38 weeks, when she went into labor and delivered Abbie, who was very sick and almost didn't make it. Abbie was born with group-B streptococcus, an infection she contracted as she passed through Nettie's birth canal.

Nettie explained to Andi that she had no warning; she hadn't been sick, she hadn't even had a discharge and had no clue that something might be wrong. She had been traveling and had missed her last two prenatal visits. She hadn't thought it mattered much.

(continued on next page)

- A culture may not always identify a woman who is colonized at the time of delivery. Cultures may be negative, and the woman later becomes colonized.
- The Centers for Disease Control, the American College of Obstetricians and Gynecologists and the

(continued from previous page)

Andi had questions and was glad she had a prenatal appointment on Monday. Her doctor had mentioned that she would have a pelvic exam at her next visit, and she hadn't been happy about it.

In the exam room on Monday, before she could ask her questions, Andi's doctor explained that during the pelvic exam she would do a culture for GBS. She said that as many as 1 in 5 (20%) of all women are positive for GBS, even though they have no symptoms. They don't have a discharge, and they aren't sick. Still the bacteria can be in the birth canal.

The doctor further explained that if the culture was positive, Andi would not receive antibiotics at that time but would get them during labor to protect the baby. Even after her appointment, Andi was still a little confused. She was glad to receive a booklet from the nurse and anxious to go home and look at her pregnancy books. She was also reassured to know that now her visits would be every week so that any problems she might have could be taken care of.

American Academy of Pediatrics have developed recommendations aimed at preventing GBS infection in newborns.

- One recommendation is that a GBS culture be taken from the rectal and vaginal areas of all pregnant women at 35 to 37 weeks of pregnancy.

- Another recommendation is that all women who have risk factors be treated for GBS.
- Risk factors for developing GBS include the following:
  - ~ a previous infant with GBS infection
  - ~ preterm labor
  - ~ ruptured membranes for more than 18 hours
  - ~ preterm/premature rupture of the membranes (before 37 weeks)
  - ~ a temperature of 100.4F immediately before or during childbirth

Ultrasound in the 3rd Trimester

If you have an ultrasound exam in the 3rd trimester, your doctor is looking for particular information. Performed later in pregnancy, this test can:

- evaluate the baby's size and growth
- determine the cause of vaginal bleeding
- check for intrauterine-growth restriction
- determine the cause of vaginal or abdominal pain
- evaluate a baby after an accident or injury to the mother-to-be
- detect some fetal malformations
- monitor the growth of multiples
- monitor a high-risk pregnancy

- measure the amount of amniotic fluid
- check the presentation of baby (breech or head-first)
- determine which delivery method to use
- determine maturity of the placenta
- determine fetal lung maturity, when used with amniocentesis
- provide reassurance of fetal well-being, when used as part of a biophysical profile

Home Uterine Monitoring

- Some women are monitored at home during pregnancy with *home uterine monitoring.*
- Contractions of a pregnant woman's uterus are recorded once or more during the day, then transmitted by telephone to the doctor or a nurse for evaluation.
- The procedure is used to identify women at risk of premature labor.
- Costs vary but run between $80 and $100 a day.

Kick Count

- Toward the end of pregnancy, you may be asked to record how often you feel your baby move.

Kick Counts Count When Baby Doesn't Move Much

This pregnancy was different for Helen. Bertha had been active in the uterus, almost tormenting her mom. She moved so much, sometimes it was annoying. Helen's clothes jumped embarrassingly, and it seemed that when Helen wanted to rest or sleep, it was playtime for baby!

Eli and Helen had assumed their second pregnancy would be more of the same, but it wasn't. This baby wasn't a mover. At 34 weeks, they had already been to labor and delivery five times to check on baby. They were more embarrassed each time, despite the reassurance the nurses gave them that their visits were OK.

Helen had tried everything—shaking her tummy with her hands, eating frequent snacks, even drinking soft drinks with caffeine—and still this baby didn't move much. Her doctor explained that there was a test Helen could do at home to help reassure them, and it might even save some trips to the hospital.

Helen started recording kick counts. She could choose when to do the test, but after eating a meal was a good time because this baby was more active then. Helen and Eli decided to do the test every day. They knew they would probably still be making some trips to the hospital but hopefully not as many.

- Done at home, this is called a *kick count.*
- A kick count provides reassurance about fetal well-being; this information is similar to that learned by a nonstress test. See the discussion of the nonstress test on page 62.

- Your doctor may use one of two common methods.
- The first method is to count how many times the baby moves in an hour.
- The second method is to note how long it takes baby to move 10 times.
- Usually you can choose when you want to do the test.
- After eating a meal is a good time to count kicks because baby is often more active then.

Bishop Score

The *Bishop score* is a method of evaluating the cervix and is used to predict the success of inducing labor. See page 97 for further information on inducing labor.

- A Bishop score is determined by several measurements, including dilatation, effacement, station, consistency and position of the cervix.
- Your doctor will make these evaluations and give you a score of 0, 1, 2 or 3 for each area, then the scores are added together.
- The total score helps predict the success of inducing labor.
- A score of 9 or higher indicates a high chance of a successful induction of active labor.
- As the Bishop score decreases, the rate for successfully inducing labor falls.

The Nonstress Test (NST) Offers Valuable Information

The name of the test didn't make much sense to Celia and Lane, but the doctor said she needed a nonstress test after she was involved in a car accident. She was tired from a long day at work, and at 35 weeks, her energy didn't last long. All Celia wanted to do was go home and go to bed.

Lane met Celia at the scene of the rear-end collision, grateful to find her OK. The car was another story, probably totaled. Fortunately Celia was wearing her seat belt, even though it was getting more difficult to do as she got bigger.

She told Lane she felt OK. She did have a few friction burns on her arms and neck from the air bag, and her tummy was tightening a little. Lane had already called their OB doctor on his cell phone, who told them he would call the hospital and advise them they were coming. An ambulance took Celia to the hospital, with Lane following in his car.

At the hospital, preliminary vital signs, including Celia's blood pressure and pulse, were taken, and a fetal monitor was put on her tummy. She had never seen a monitor before but had seen pictures of one in her childbirth-education class a few weeks ago.

When the labor nurse plugged in the cord, Celia could hear the sound of her baby's heart racing along. "Is it too fast? Is it all right?" She was worried by all the attention she was getting, especially when they started an I.V.

The nurse smiled and replied, "It looks good. We need to monitor you for a while, then we'll do a nonstress test." She told Celia and Lane babies are well protected inside the uterus, and the amniotic fluid provides good protection in an accident.

(continued on next page)

(continued from previous page)

The nurse went on to explain that the nonstress test gave information about the baby's condition.

The nurse handed Celia a button with a cord connected to the monitor machine. She instructed Celia to push the button every time the baby moved, which would make a mark on the monitor paper. With a good test (reactive), the baby's heartbeat would increase 10 to 15 beats when it moved. With a poor test (nonreactive or nonreassuring), baby's heartbeat didn't change with movement. She further explained that a nonreactive or nonreassuring nonstress test didn't mean something was wrong; it just wasn't reassuring.

Celia did as she was instructed and pushed the button every time she felt the baby move. Results were reassuring, and she was sent home a few hours later. As Lane and Celia drove home, they both admitted they had been a little worried about their baby but now felt better after having the test.

Nonstress Test (NST)

A *nonstress test* (NST) is a simple, noninvasive procedure done at 32 weeks of pregnancy or later.

- The test is performed in the doctor's office or in the labor-and-delivery department at the hospital.
- It measures the response of the fetal heart to movement and evaluates fetal well-being in late pregnancy.
- Doctors use the findings from the NST to help them evaluate how well a baby is tolerating life inside the uterus.

- The nonstress test is commonly used in overdue and high-risk pregnancies.
- The test takes from 10 minutes to 45 minutes to complete.
- While you are lying down, a technician attaches a fetal monitor (Doppler ultrasound) to your abdomen.
- Every time you feel your baby move, you push a button to make a mark on a strip of monitor paper. At the same time, the monitor records the baby's heartbeat.
- When the baby moves, its heart rate usually goes up.
- If the baby doesn't move or if the heart rate does not react to movement, the test is called *nonreactive.*
- When baby doesn't move, it doesn't necessarily mean there is a problem—the baby may be sleeping.
- To help make baby move, you may be given something to eat or drink.
- If the baby still doesn't move, a buzzer that creates a sound and vibration to wake up the fetus may be used to make it move. This is called *vibration stimulation.*
- A nonreactive test might be a sign the baby is not receiving enough oxygen or is experiencing some other problem. However, in more than 75% of nonreactive tests, the baby is healthy.
- If your test is nonreactive, the test will probably be repeated in 24 hours or additional tests may be or-

dered, including a contraction-stress test or a biophysical profile.

- Your doctor will decide if further action is necessary. See the discussions that follow.

Contraction-Stress Test (CST)

If your nonstress test is nonreactive (see the previous discussion), a *contraction-stress test* (CST), also called a *stress test*, may be ordered.

- The contraction-stress test measures the response of the fetal heart to mild uterine contractions that mimic labor.
- It also gives an indication of how the baby is doing and how well the baby might tolerate contractions and labor.
- Some believe the CST is more accurate than the nonstress test in evaluating a baby's well-being.
- If you have had a problem pregnancy in the past or if you experienced medical problems during this pregnancy, your doctor may order this test in the last few weeks of pregnancy.
- If you have diabetes and take insulin, your baby may be at some increased risk of problems. In that situation, the test may be done every week, beginning around 32 weeks.

- In some cases, the doctor may order the nonstress test alone or order both the nonstress test and the contraction-stress test at the same time.
- A contraction-stress test is usually done in the hospital because it occasionally triggers labor.
- A monitor is placed on your abdomen to record the fetal heart rate.

When Is the Contraction-Stress Test (CST) Done?

Marti's diabetes hadn't been a problem during her pregnancy. Her doctor had told her and James at their first prenatal visit several months ago it was a very good thing she had taken such good care of herself before her pregnancy and her diabetes was under control.

They were a little surprised to learn that women with diabetes had often had difficult pregnancies years ago. These women had been at increased risk for complications and birth defects, and many had Cesarean deliveries. The doctor explained during their first visit that beginning at about 32 weeks, Marti would have some tests to keep an eye on the baby.

By 37 weeks, Marti had had a nonstress test every week for 5 weeks; they were getting to be routine. That was until the day she had been in such a hurry she had skipped breakfast and hadn't eaten very much during the day. She felt awful. She called the doctor, and he advised her to have another nonstress test.

(continued on next page)

(continued from previous page)

The nurses had been trying to get a reassuring result for about an hour. They had given Marti juice to drink and even used a little buzzer/vibrator on her tummy in an attempt to wake up the baby and get it to move.

Unsuccessful, they said her doctor wanted her to have a stress test, short for contraction-stress test or CST. It wasn't that the nonstress test was a poor test; the test results just weren't reassuring. The nurse explained they would need to make Marti's uterus contract, then, using the monitor, they could see if the baby was all right.

Marti was told that there were two ways to make her uterus contract. One was with a medication, oxytocin, in an I.V. The other way was using nipple stimulation. Marti thought this was a joke at first. However, the nurse explained that by rolling her nipple gently between her fingers, it could make her uterus contract.

Marti decided to try the nipple stimulation first and was glad it worked. It really wasn't that bad, and she didn't need the I.V. Her test visit had been longer than usual, but Marti and James were glad of the reassurance they received when the CST showed the baby was fine.

- You will be attached to an I.V. that dispenses small amounts of the hormone oxytocin to make your uterus contract, or nipple stimulation may be used to make your uterus contract.
- Three contractions must be recorded in about 10 minutes, and each contraction must last about 40 seconds. The entire test can take as long as 2 hours.

- The baby's heartbeat is monitored for its response to the contractions.
- When your uterus contracts, the blood flow to the placenta decreases.
- If the baby is having trouble or the placenta isn't working well, the contraction can decrease the oxygen supply to the baby. This causes the fetal heart rate to drop.
- The results of the test can be classified as *negative, positive, unsatisfactory* or *equivocal.*
- A negative test is good. A positive test is not good. Unsatisfactory or equivocal results mean the test was neither positive nor negative.
- Test results can indicate how well a baby might tolerate contractions and labor.
- If the baby doesn't respond well to contractions, it can be a sign of fetal stress.
- A slowed heart rate after a contraction may be a sign of fetal stress.
- Your doctor may recommend delivery of the baby, if the CST is not reassuring.
- In other cases, the test may be repeated the next day, or a biophysical profile may be ordered. (See the discussion beginning on page 69.)
- If the test shows no sign of a slowed fetal heart rate, the test result is reassuring.

The Biophysical Profile

A *biophysical profile* is an in-depth test to examine the baby during the last 2 months of pregnancy. It is a non-stress test combined with ultrasound evaluations.

- A biophysical profile helps determine fetal health and is done when there is need for reassurance about the baby or there is concern about fetal well-being.
- The test is usually done in high-risk situations, overdue pregnancies or pregnancies in which the baby doesn't move very much.
- It's also useful in evaluating an infant with intrauterine-growth restriction.
- The test takes 30 to 40 minutes.
- A biophysical profile uses a particular scoring system. A score is given to each of the five areas of evaluation listed below; the first four of the five tests are made with ultrasound; the fifth is done with external fetal monitors.
- Fetal breathing movements—Fetal "breathing" involves the movement or expansion of the baby's chest inside the uterus. This score is based on the amount of movement that occurs.
- Fetal body movements—Movement of the baby's body is noted. A normal score indicates normal body movements. An abnormal score is given when

there are few or no body movements during the allotted time period.

- Fetal tone—Fetal tone is evaluated similarly. Movement, or lack of movement, of the arms and legs of the baby is rated.
- Amount of amniotic fluid—Evaluation of the amount of amniotic fluid requires experience in ultrasound examination. A normal pregnancy has adequate fluid around the baby. An abnormal test indicates little or no amniotic fluid around the baby.
- Reactive fetal heart rate—Fetal heart-rate monitoring (nonstress test) is done with external monitors. It evaluates changes in the fetal heart rate associated with movement of the baby. The amount of change and number of changes in the fetal heart rate can differ, depending on who is doing the test and their definition of normal.
- Evaluation may vary depending on the sophistication of the equipment used and the expertise of the person doing the test.
- For each test, a normal score is 2; an abnormal score is 0. A score of 1 in any of the tests is a middle score.
- From these five scores, a total score is obtained by adding all the values together.
- The higher the score, the better the baby's condition. A lower score may cause concern about the well-being of the fetus.

The Biophysical Profile—A Comprehensive Test

Mike and Wendi had grown weary of tests. When their doctor first discussed the various tests Wendi might have, they were happy for the reassurances they would get. Their first pregnancy had ended in disaster—their baby died at 38 weeks of pregnancy without any warning.

They decided this pregnancy was going well. They were very frightened at first but relaxed more as the pregnancy progressed.

The close monitoring had begun with a few extra blood tests in the 1st trimester, then an extra ultrasound in the 2nd trimester. Starting at 32 weeks, Wendi had weekly nonstress tests; it had become boring.

Now in the last month, the testing was more involved and took more time. Her doctor told Wendi she wanted her to have a biophysical profile. As it had been explained to them, five tests would be done—fetal breathing movements, fetal body movements, fetal tone, amount of amniotic fluid and a nonstress test.

The five areas were each scored 0, 1 or 2; the higher the better. The scores were totaled; a low score could raise concern about the well-being of the fetus. The tests 2 days ago had resulted in a score that was lower than last week's test.

The couple had been instructed to return yet again for another biophysical profile. "Is it really necessary to spend all that time at the hospital again? I shouldn't miss work again today," Mike had said this morning. Wendi had felt like agreeing, but today the baby hadn't been moving as much as she was used to, and it worried her.

When the monitor was put on Wendi's abdomen, it showed she was having mild contractions that she couldn't feel. The baby's heartbeat on the monitor looked different—flatter and

(continued on next page)

(continued from previous page)

smoother. When Wendi had a contraction, the baby's heartbeat dropped and slowed down.

Things happened quickly. They tried to start her labor, but the baby's heartbeat got worse. Wendi's doctor decided to do an emergency Cesarean section.

Afterward, the couple was together in recovery, admiring their beautiful daughter. The biophysical profile testing had helped them avoid another disaster.

- A score of 8 to 10 is reassuring; 4 or less is not reassuring.
- If the score is low, a recommendation may be made to deliver the baby.
- If the score is reassuring, the test may be repeated at a later date.
- If results fall in the middle, the test may be repeated the following day, depending on the circumstances of the pregnancy and the findings of the biophysical profile.

Tests You May Have during Labor

Labor Check

- If you think you may be in labor and go to the hospital, you will have a *labor check.*

- Vital signs will be taken, a monitor will be placed on your abdomen and a pelvic exam will be performed.
- These tests are done to determine if you are in labor and if your pregnancy is doing OK.
- If you are not in labor, you will be given instructions and sent home. Your instructions will include precautions and warning signs.
- No one wants to be sent home, but it is OK. You'll be back soon.

Fetal Blood Sampling during Labor

Fetal blood sampling helps to evaluate how well a baby tolerates the stress of labor.

- Before the test can be performed, your membranes must be ruptured (your water has broken), and the cervix must be dilated at least 2cm (about an inch).
- Once you are dilated to 2cm, an instrument is passed into the vagina, through the dilated cervix, to the top of the baby's head, where it makes a small nick in the baby's scalp.
- The baby's blood is collected in a small tube, and its pH (acidity) is checked.
- The baby's pH level indicates whether the baby is having trouble or is under stress.

- The test helps the doctor decide whether labor can continue or if a Cesarean delivery is needed.

Fetal Monitoring (Electronic Fetal Monitoring)

In many hospitals, a baby's heartbeat is monitored throughout labor with external fetal monitoring or internal fetal monitoring. A normal fetal heart rate is from 110 to 160 beats a minute.

- *External fetal monitoring* can be done before your membranes rupture (water breaks).
- A pair of belts are strapped to your abdomen to record your contractions and the baby's heartbeat.
- One strap holds an ultrasound to monitor fetal heart rate. The other strap holds a device to measure the length of contractions and how often they occur.
- *Internal fetal monitoring* monitors the baby more precisely.
- An electrode, called a *scalp electrode,* is placed through the vagina then attached to the fetus's scalp to measure the fetal heart rate.
- A thin tube, called an *internal pressure catheter,* can be put inside the uterus to monitor the strength of the contractions.
- This is done *only* after membranes have ruptured.

- It may be a little uncomfortable to have monitors placed or inserted, but it is not painful.
- Monitors send information to a machine that records the information on a strip of paper.
- Results can usually be seen in your room and at the nurses' station. In some places, your doctor can check results on his or her computer.
- In most cases, when you are monitored, you must stay in bed. In some places, wireless monitors are available so you can move around.

Fetal Monitoring during Labor

Her friends had warned Eloise about fetal monitoring. A few had advised her to refuse it, saying, "It is too invasive, it causes C-sections and it can hurt your baby." Others had said that it wasn't so bad; they were actually glad their baby's condition could be checked while they were in labor.

When her time came, Eloise and Larry had rushed to the hospital in the middle of the night and discovered she was in early labor. They had walked for an hour and a half in the hospital to see if her labor would get going. She knew that something was happening—in the last half hour she had had to stop to breathe through the contractions, which were quite painful.

When she got back into bed for the nurses to do a labor check, Eloise had gone from 1cm to 3cm. As the nurse was placing an external monitor on her abdomen, Eloise asked her about it. The nurse explained that the monitor kept track of her contractions

(continued on next page)

(continued from previous page)

and her baby's heartbeat. She said that both helped the nurses and Eloise's doctor make sure her baby was doing OK with labor.

Eloise decided it sounded like a good idea, but she wanted to ask another question. "Do monitors cause more C-sections to happen?" Her nurse smiled and reassured Eloise that wasn't the purpose of the monitor. However, monitoring could help identify those babies in trouble that might need a quick delivery (by C-section) or other treatment during labor. She said the fetal heart monitor worked using a principle similar to ultrasound, and the contraction monitor worked by a pressure sensor on her abdomen. The nurse further reassured her that the information on the screen in her room was viewed at the nurses' station, and in some instances, her doctor could also check the tracing on his computer at home or in the office.

A few hours later the doctor came into her room. He explained they were having trouble keeping track of the baby with the external monitor and believed an internal monitor would give better information. With an internal monitor, a small wire is attached to the baby's skin to provide a continuous recording of the fetal heart rate. Placement of the monitor would rupture her membranes (break her water). He said they might want to place another internal monitor (an intrauterine pressure catheter) to better evaluate her contractions. This type of monitor is a small tube, similar to a small straw, that slides next to the baby's head inside the uterus.

Eloise had been at the hospital for 12 hours, and her cervix had stopped dilating and changing. She was ready for anything! Eloise and Larry were happy to learn these devices were available to safeguard their baby during labor. And Eloise was happy when the doctor told her the anesthesiologist was on his way.

Evaluating Fetal Lung Maturity

The respiratory system is the last fetal system to mature. Premature infants often have respiratory difficulties because their lungs are not fully developed.

- Knowing how mature a baby's lungs are helps in deciding about early delivery, if that must be considered.
- If the baby needs to be delivered early, tests can predict whether the baby will be able to breathe without assistance.
- There are several fetal lung maturity tests available, including:
  - lecithin/sphingomyelin ratio (L/S ratio)
  - phosphatidyl glycerol (PG)
  - foam stability index
  - fluorescence polarization
  - optical density at 650nm
  - lamellar body counts
  - saturated phosphatidylcholine
- The test done depends on availability and the experience of those taking care of the pregnant woman.
- Two tests used most often to evaluate a baby's lungs before birth are the *L/S ratio* and the *phosphatidyl glycerol* (PG) tests.
- Fluid for these two tests is obtained by amniocentesis.

Test to Determine Baby's Oxygen Levels

- We can now monitor baby's oxygen *inside* the womb, before birth.
- This test, called *OxiFirst* fetal oxygen monitoring, is used during labor.
- This test is not available everywhere, but studies have shown the test increases the effectiveness of fetal-heart monitors.
- Oxygen levels are measured by placing a sensor through the birth canal and attaching it to the baby's cheek.
- Light measures the oxygen level in fetal blood, providing accurate answers as to whether baby's oxygen levels are in the safe range.
- If an abnormal heart rate is found—this occurs in 30% of all births where monitors are used—oxygen levels can be helpful in determining whether a C- section should be performed.
- If low levels are detected, decisions can be made about delivering the baby.

Inducing Labor

There may come a point in your pregnancy when you and your doctor decide to induce labor for your health or the health of your baby. This is a fairly common practice—each year, doctors in the U.S. induce labor for about 450,000 births.

- Labor is induced for overdue babies, but it is also used for a number of other reasons, including chronic high blood pressure in the mother-to-be, ruptured membranes without contractions, pre-eclampsia, gestational diabetes, intrauterine-growth restriction and Rh-isoimmunization.
- When you see the doctor late in pregnancy, you will probably have a pelvic exam.
- This may also include an evaluation of how ready you are for an induction.
- Your doctor may use the Bishop score to help make this determination (see page 61). See also the discussion of inducing labor in the section on page 78.

Tests for Your Newborn

Immediately and shortly after baby's birth, your new baby will be given many tests in the hospital. These tests help determine your baby's health and may reveal problems that need to be dealt with. They also provide the pediatrician with information about any potential problems. Your newborn will be observed for:

- unusual skin color
- temperature-control problems (high or low)
- change in activity
- cardiac and respiratory rate and rhythm
- abnormalities of the stool
- problems urinating
- excessive sleepiness or lethargy
- abdominal bloating
- most babies are also tested for hearing problems and eye problems before they are released

Apgar Score

- This test was developed by Virginia Apgar, M.D., and is used to assess your newborn's overall condition immediately after birth.
- The baby is evaluated at 1 minute and 5 minutes after birth; a score of 0, 1 or 2 is possible in five areas—heart rate, color, muscle tone, respiratory effort and reflex irritability.
- For each test, scores from the five criteria are added together, for a maximum total of 10.
- An average score for most normal, healthy babies is 7 to 9.

- The Apgar score is used to determine the baby's current health following delivery but is not used to predict future health.

Blood Tests

- Shortly after delivery, blood is taken from baby's heel for a blood screen.
- Tests are done on the blood for many problems, including the following:
  - ~ anemia
  - ~ hypothyroidism
  - ~ sickle-cell anemia
  - ~ blood-glucose levels
- Results often indicate whether baby needs further evaluation.

Coombs Test

- The Coombs test is administered if the mother's blood is Rh-negative, Type O or if the mother has not been tested for antibodies.
- It tests blood taken from the umbilical cord.
- Test results indicate whether Rh-antibodies have been formed.

Reflex Assessment

- The reflex assessment tests for several specific reflexes in baby, including the rooting and grasp reflexes.
- If a particular reflex is not observed, further evaluation will be done.

Neonatal Maturity Assessment

- In this test, various characteristics of baby are assessed to evaluate baby's neuromuscular and physical maturity.
- Like the Apgar test, each characteristic is assigned a score, and the sum indicates baby's maturity.

Brazelton Neonatal Behavioral Assessment Scale

- This test covers a broad range of newborn behavior.
- It is also an observation test and provides information about how a newborn responds to his or her environment.
- The test is usually used when a problem is suspected, but some hospitals test all babies.

Other Newborn Tests

Most states offer other routine screening tests for newborns, including:

- biotinidase—to determine if the baby is deficient in this essential enzyme
- congenital adrenal hyperplasia—to learn if the adrenal glands are functioning properly
- congenital hypothyroidism—to check thyroid hormone levels
- cystic fibrosis—to determine if the baby has cystic fibrosis
- hemoglobinopathies—to check for defects in the hemoglobin
- homocysteinuria—to learn if a baby has a B_{12} deficiency and a special diet is necessary
- galactosemia—to determine if the baby can handle galactose efficiently
- maple-syrup urine disease—to determine if some amino acids must be restricted for baby
- PKU—to test for phenylketonuria, a metabolic disease
- In February, 1998, New York became the first state to require hospitals to check every newborn for HIV. Results are reported to the mother or guardian.

Your After-Pregnancy Checkup

Your postpartum (after-birth) checkup is the last part of your complete prenatal-care program. This appointment is as important as any during your pregnancy, so don't miss it!

- A postpartum checkup is scheduled between 2 and 6 weeks after delivery, depending on whether you had a Cesarean delivery or a vaginal delivery, or if you had any problems.
- At your visit, your doctor will want to hear how you feel.
- Be sure to write down any questions about getting back on your feet, and take them with you so you can remember them all.
- This visit is also a good time to discuss birth control, if you haven't already made plans.
- A complete blood count (CBC) may be done to check your iron stores and to check for infections, especially if you lost a lot of blood during the birth.
- If you have had headaches or experienced increased irritability or fatigue, your doctor may prescribe an iron supplement.
- You may also have a physical exam, similar to the one at your first prenatal exam. If this is the case,

you may need to schedule more time. Ask about it when you make your appointment.

- Part of the physical will be a pelvic exam. If you had any birth tears or incisions, your doctor will examine them to see how they are healing.
- A pelvic exam is also done to determine if your uterus is returning to its prepregnant size and position.
- You may also have a Pap smear. If your Pap test reveals an infection, it will be treated.
- If your Pap smear was abnormal before or at the beginning of your pregnancy, the test will be done again at this time.
- Women who deliver vaginally may see a change in abnormal Pap smears; they may become normal. One study showed that 60% of a group of women who had problem Pap smears before birth had normal Pap smears after their baby was born.
- If the test reveals a precancerous condition, called *dysplasia,* the next step is usually a colposcopy. With a colposcopy, a microscope is used to examine your cervix and to look for abnormal areas. If any are found, a sample of the tissue is removed, called a *biopsy.* This can be done now that you are not pregnant.

Do You Need a Pap Smear and Pelvic Exam after Delivery?

When she made the appointment for her 6-week postpartum exam, Phoebe thought she'd find an excuse to miss the appointment. She didn't want to keep it. When she'd had a Pap smear and pelvic exam at the beginning of pregnancy, her doctor had said her Pap smear wasn't normal. In fact, the result was precancerous, and if she hadn't been pregnant, a biopsy would have been recommended.

The doctor had done a colposcopy (without biopsy) during the pregnancy because of the abnormal test result. In the hospital, she had impressed upon Phoebe how important it was for her to have another Pap smear after the pregnancy, so Phoebe reluctantly kept the postpartum appointment.

The 6-week exam hadn't been that bad; it was fun to see her friends in the office again and to show off her new baby. Even seeing the doctor was enjoyable.

A week later, Phoebe was on hold waiting for the doctor to give her the results of her Pap smear. She was nervous. However, she was surprised, happy and confused when her doctor told her that her Pap smear from her 6-week exam was normal.

The doctor reminded Phoebe that she had explained to her following the abnormal test result several months ago that pregnancy can change abnormal Pap smears. It isn't unusual for an abnormal Pap smear result in early pregnancy to change to normal after pregnancy. Phoebe listened as her doctor explained how her cervix had stretched and dilated during labor, then shrunk back to normal afterward. In effect, the cervix was traumatized then healed. The irregular cells causing the abnormal Pap smear were also healed in the process. It wasn't always bad news when your doctor called, Phoebe thought with a smile!

Hematocrit

In some cases, a hematocrit (Hct) test will be done at your 6-week visit. A hematocrit test is part of a complete blood count (CBC).

- The Hct measures the percentage of your blood that is made up of cells.
- A similar evaluation is the hemoglobin level of the blood, which is the part of the blood that carries oxygen from the lungs to the other tissues of the body.
- Hematocrit and hemoglobin levels are used to determine if you have anemia.
- Anemia is any condition in which the number of red blood cells and/or the hemoglobin level are less than normal.
- Childbirth, surgery, such as a C-section, or bleeding a lot after baby's birth can lead to anemia because of blood loss.
- If you have anemia, you may be given iron to treat it.

Part II: Medical Procedures during Pregnancy

Various medical procedures are done during pregnancy to ensure your health and the health of your baby. The discussions that follow outline what procedures your doctor might want to discuss with you, depending on problems you may encounter. Knowing about them helps you prepare questions to ask and helps you make decisions so you can actively participate in your care.

Maternal Procedures during Pregnancy

McDonald's Cerclage for an Incompetent Cervix

- An *incompetent cervix* is a condition in which a woman's cervix dilates (stretches) prematurely, without contractions or pain. Usually the woman doesn't notice the condition because it isn't painful.
- With an incompetent cervix, your membranes may rupture (your water breaks) without warning and your baby will usually be delivered prematurely.
- An incompetent cervix is not usually diagnosed until after one or more deliveries of a premature infant without any pain before delivery.

- If you have already had a premature baby and an incompetent cervix is determined to have been the problem, your doctor may check your cervix for competency during your next pregnancy.
- If this is your first pregnancy, you cannot know if you have an incompetent cervix.
- Some researchers believe the condition may occur because of previous trauma to the cervix, such as a miscarriage.
- It may also occur if surgery has previously been performed on the cervix.
- Once your doctor detects a weak cervix, he or she can reinforce it by sewing the cervix shut. This procedure is called a *McDonald's cerclage* or *cervical cerclage.*
- This procedure is usually performed early in the 2nd trimester, most often between weeks 14 and 16. It can be done up to 24 weeks.
- A McDonald's cerclage is usually performed in a hospital operating room or in labor and delivery.
- General anesthesia or I.V. sedation is given.
- A suture, similar to a "purse-string," is stitched around the cervix to keep it closed.
- The procedure takes about 30 minutes.
- Usually you will be monitored for a few hours afterward, then go home.

- It is normal to have a little bit of spotting or bleeding afterward.
- At about 36 weeks or when you go into labor, the stitch is removed, and baby can be born normally.
- The suture is removed in labor and delivery without anesthesia. It takes about 5 minutes.
- Labor does not necessarily happen right after it is removed; it can occur in a few days to a few weeks.

Rh-Sensitivity and RhoGAM

We have discussed the blood tests you will have early in your pregnancy. These tests have determined your blood type and Rh-factor.

- The *Rh-factor* is a protein in the blood; it is determined by a genetic trait.
- If you are Rh-positive, it means you have the factor; *Rh-negative* means the factor is missing. Being Rh-negative is not as common as being Rh-positive.
- If you are Rh-positive, you don't have to worry about any of this.
- If you are Rh-negative and your baby is, too, there is no problem.
- But if you are Rh-negative and your baby is Rh-positive, it's a situation you need to know about.

- If you are Rh-negative and your baby is Rh-positive or if you have had a blood transfusion or received blood products of some kind, there's a risk you could become Rh-sensitized or isoimmunized.
- *Isoimmunized* means you have made antibodies that circulate inside your system; they don't harm you but can cross the placenta and get into your baby's circulation. These antibodies are directed against Rh-positive blood and can attack the Rh-positive blood of your growing baby. This situation can cause blood disease of the fetus or newborn, and it can make your baby anemic while it is still inside your uterus.
- Fortunately, this reaction is preventable. The use of Rh-immune globulin (RhoGAM) has alleviated many problems.
- RhoGAM is a product that is extracted from human blood. It prevents your immune system from recognizing the foreign Rh-positive blood in your system. This prevents you from forming antibodies to Rh-positive blood.
- If you are Rh-negative and your baby is Rh-positive, your doctor may give you a shot of RhoGAM at 28 weeks of pregnancy to prevent sensitization before delivery.
- An injection of RhoGAM may also be given to you if you are exposed to your baby's blood, which is

more likely to happen during the last 3 months of pregnancy and at delivery. This can happen with a fall, an accident or when you have contractions.

- RhoGAM is also given to you within 72 hours after delivery, if your baby is Rh-positive.
- You may also be given multiple doses of RhoGAM following your baby's delivery if blood tests show that a larger than normal number of Rh-positive blood cells (from your baby) have entered your bloodstream. This is determined by testing your blood shortly after baby's delivery.
- The blood test to determine how much fetal blood may have gotten into your circulation system is called a *Kleihauer-Betke test.* The Kleihauer-Betke test can determine if more than one dose of RhoGAM needs to be given.
- If your baby is Rh-negative, you don't need RhoGAM after delivery and you didn't need the shot during pregnancy. But it's better not to take that risk and to have the RhoGAM injection during pregnancy. You will not know your baby's blood type during pregnancy unless you have amniocentesis.
- If you have an ectopic pregnancy and are Rh-negative, you should receive RhoGAM. This applies to miscarriages and abortions as well.

Are You Rh-Negative?

Shelley and Bart asked a lot of questions about the tests Shelley had had early in her pregnancy. She was surprised to find out that she was Rh-negative; her blood type was O-negative. Bart knew his blood type was O-positive from being tested in the military.

The doctor assured them this wasn't anything to worry about. From her blood work, the doctor also told Shelley she was "antibody negative." This means she had not already made antibodies to Rh-positive blood, which was good. Her doctor explained that she could become "antibody positive" (make antibodies to Rh-positive blood) during pregnancy or during delivery, or from a blood transfusion of Rh-positive blood.

Now at 28 weeks, the doctor wanted to do another blood test to check for antibodies. If Shelley was still negative for antibodies to Rh-positive blood, they would give her a shot of RhoGAM. The RhoGAM would protect her until she delivered in case Rh-positive blood got into her circulation from her baby. If she had antibodies, she had become sensitized or isoimmunized and would be treated for that condition.

After Bozo (their pregnancy name for baby) was born, his blood type would also be checked. If he was Rh-positive, Shelley would get more RhoGAM to prevent her from making antibodies against Rh-positive blood. This could make a difference in future pregnancies. If Bozo's blood type was Rh-negative, Shelley would not need any more RhoGAM, and she hadn't needed the shot she got at 28 weeks.

It all sounded very technical and confusing to Bart and Shelley. They were reassured that years ago being Rh-negative could seriously complicate a pregnancy, but now that we understand what to do and have RhoGAM available, it rarely causes a problem today.

- If any invasive procedures are done during your pregnancy that may cause the baby's blood to mix with yours, such as amniocentesis or chorionic villus sampling, and you are Rh-negative, you should receive RhoGAM.
- Some women have expressed concern about the risk of contracting hepatitis or HIV from use of RhoGAM, but problems have not been reported. Donors for Rh-immune globulin are screened carefully to eliminate those in high-risk groups for transmission of infectious diseases. If you are concerned, talk with your doctor.
- If you have religious, ethical or personal reasons for not using blood or blood products, consult your physician or minister.

Fetal Procedures and Surgeries

Today, we are truly fortunate to be able to take care of some fetal problems *before* a baby is born. In the past, we had to wait until after baby's birth to deal with them. Now, we can correct some of them so a baby is born healthy, with little impact on his or her long-term health.

- Surgeries treat a variety of fetal problems, including urinary-tract blockages, tumors and fluid in the lungs.
- Sometimes a baby needs a blood transfusion shortly after birth. In severe cases, transfusions are done *before* the baby is born.
- There are two kinds of fetal surgeries—open surgery and closed-uterus surgery.
- Most surgeries, whether open or closed-uterus, are not performed until at least the 28th week of pregnancy.

Open Surgery

- With open surgery (first done in 1981), the surgeon makes a Cesareanlike incision in the mother's abdomen and uterus.
- The fetus is partially removed from the uterus. Surgery is performed as necessary, then the fetus is returned to the uterus.
- Performing open surgery on a fetus means that a mother will later have to have a Cesarean to deliver her baby.
- This kind of surgery carries risks for both mother and baby.

- One problem with open surgery is that it may stimulate uterine contractions, which can lead to premature birth.
- In addition, it exposes the mother to all the risks of surgery, including anesthesia problems, bleeding and infections.

Closed-Uterus Surgery

- Closed-uterus procedures are more common than open surgeries.
- With this surgery, a needle-thin, fiber-optic instrument is guided by miniature cameras inside the abdomen and uterus into the fetus's body while the fetus remains inside the womb.
- The necessary corrective procedure is performed while the fetus is still inside the uterus. This procedure poses fewer risks to the baby and mother.
- The most successful closed-uterus surgeries are those that deal with opening blocked urinary tracts.

Inducing Labor

There may come a point late in your pregnancy when your doctor decides to induce labor; it's a fairly common practice. Labor is induced for overdue babies, chronic high blood pressure in the mother, pre-eclampsia, gestational diabetes, intrauterine-growth restriction and Rh-isoimmunization. Each year, U.S. doctors induce labor for about 450,000 births. Inducing labor usually happens after the 36th week of pregnancy and through to postterm pregnancies.

- While the fetus is growing and developing inside your uterus, it depends on two important functions performed by the placenta—respiration and nutrition—for growth and development.
- When a baby is overdue, the placenta may not provide the respiratory function or essential nutrients the baby needs to grow, and an infant may begin to suffer nutritional deprivation. The baby is called *postmature.*
- A pregnancy is considered to be overdue (*postterm*) only when it exceeds 42 weeks or 294 days from the first day of the last menstrual period. (A baby that is 41 weeks and 6 days is *not* postterm!)
- If you are overdue, your doctor may examine you to determine if the baby is moving around in the womb and if the amount of amniotic fluid is healthy and normal. This evaluation may be done with a biophysical profile, as discussed on page 69.
- If the baby is healthy and active, you are usually monitored until labor begins on its own.

- If your doctor induces labor, you may first have your cervix ripened, as described below, then you will receive oxytocin (Pitocin) intravenously.
- This medication is gradually increased until contractions begin.
- The amount of oxytocin you receive is controlled by a pump, so you can't receive too much of it. While you receive oxytocin, you and your baby will be monitored for the baby's reaction to your labor.
- The length of the entire process—ripening your cervix until the birth of your baby—varies from woman to woman.
- It is important to realize that being induced or having an induction does *not* guarantee a vaginal delivery. In many instances, the induction doesn't work. In such cases, a C-section is usually necessary.

Ripening the Cervix for Induction

Today, doctors sometimes ripen the cervix before labor is induced. *Ripening the cervix* means medication is used to help the cervix soften, thin and dilate.

- The most common medications used for this purpose are Prepidil Gel (dinoprostone cervical gel, 0.5mg) and Cervidil (dinoprostone, 10mg).

- In most cases, doctors use Prepidil Gel or Cervidil to prepare the cervix the day before induction.
- Both preparations are placed in the top of the vagina, behind the cervix.
- Medication is released directly onto the cervix, which helps it to ripen (soften) for induction of labor.
- Doctors do this procedure in the labor-and-delivery area of the hospital, so the baby can be monitored.

Rupturing Membranes

- Rupturing membranes involves breaking the amniotic sac, which can stimulate contractions, if they haven't started, or make them stronger if they have already started.
- It is done in your hospital's labor-and-delivery area during a pelvic exam.
- Membranes are ruptured with an instrument called an *amni hook* (a thin plastic instrument the size of a straw) or by placing an internal fetal monitor on the baby's head.
- Although having a pelvic exam may be uncomfortable at this late stage of your pregnancy, rupturing membranes is not at all painful.

Stripping Membranes

- Some doctors "strip membranes" to make labor start; however, this procedure is controversial.
- Stripping membranes causes the release of hormones called *prostaglandins* that can cause contractions that lead to labor. It may cause you to bleed a little and to cramp.
- To strip your membranes, the doctor inserts a gloved hand through the vagina and inserts a finger through the cervix.
- He or she then sweeps a finger between the cervix and the fetal membranes (amniotic sac).

Anesthesia

Many women hope for labor and delivery without much pain medication or anesthesia, and a few women are successful in delivering without any medication. Other women are certain they want to have pain medication during labor, or they make the decision to ask for it when the pain of labor grows too intense. Whatever your feelings on anesthesia during labor, it is helpful to know your options before labor begins so that you can make informed choices at that time.

Epidural Block

Epidural block is a procedure done during labor to numb the pain of contractions or for a C-section.

- An epidural is usually performed by an anesthesiologist or a nurse trained in the procedure (a certified nurse anesthetist or CNA).
- To receive an epidural, you will be asked to sit up or lie on your side and to curve your spine and push your back out.
- Antiseptic solution is used to wash your back, then your skin is numbed with a local anesthetic, so the catheter can be inserted.
- A needle is placed into your middle or lower back, near the spine, into the epidural space.
- A small plastic catheter similar to an I.V. is placed in the space, and anesthetic medication is given through this catheter.
- When you need pain relief, it is given with a syringe through the catheter or the catheter is attached to a pump that gradually releases it.

Spinal Block

- A *spinal block* is similar to an epidural. It is usually used only for C-sections; it is not usually used in labor.

- A spinal is given like an epidural, but only the needle is placed into the spinal canal; no catheter is left in place.
- Medication is given through the needle, and a single dose lasts long enough for a Cesarean delivery.

General Anesthesia

- General anesthesia is usually used for emergency Cesarean deliveries, when there isn't time for an epidural or spinal block.
- It is administered using I.V. and inhaled medications.
- If you receive general anesthesia, you are unconscious or asleep.

Local Block

- A local block provides pain relief in a localized area.
- It is given in the area between the vagina and rectum using a needle and syringe.
- It is most often used just before delivery to provide pain relief for an episiotomy.

Episiotomy

An *episiotomy* is an incision made from the vagina toward the rectum during delivery. It is done to avoid tearing in the area as the baby's head passes through the birth canal.

- Having an episiotomy helps avoid stretching the vagina, bladder and rectum.
- Stretching the vagina can result in loss of control of your urine or bowels and can change sensations experienced during sexual intercourse.
- The reason for an episiotomy usually becomes clear at delivery when the baby's head is in the vagina.
- An episiotomy substitutes a controlled, straight, clean cut for a tear or rip that could go in many directions. This may include tearing or ripping into the bladder, large blood vessels or rectum.
- An episiotomy can also heal better than a ragged tear.
- Before the episiotomy cut is made, the area is usually washed with antiseptic soap and numbed with local anesthetic.
- The cut may be made in the midline toward the rectum, or it may be a cut to the side.
- Description of an episiotomy also includes a description of the depth of the incision:
  - a *first-degree* episiotomy cuts only the skin
  - a *second-degree* episiotomy cuts the skin and underlying tissue

  - a *third-degree* episiotomy cuts the skin, underlying tissue and rectal sphincter, which is the muscle that goes around the anus
  - a *fourth-degree* episiotomy goes through the three layers and through the rectal mucosa
- The most painful part of the entire birth experience might be an episiotomy, and it may cause some discomfort as it heals.
- Don't be afraid to ask for medication to ease pain. There are many medications that are safe to take, even if you breastfeed your baby.

Repair of an Episiotomy

- An episiotomy repair is done while you are meeting your new baby.
- After the baby is delivered, layers are closed separately with absorbable sutures that don't need to be removed after they heal.
- The episiotomy cut is repaired with sutures that are absorbed over the next few weeks.
- The two sides of the cut area are pulled together with a continuous suture.
- This procedure can take from 5 minutes to 1 hour.

Forceps Delivery and Vacuum Extraction

Some deliveries require assistance to help deliver the baby's head. This may occur if you push for a long time but the baby's head just won't deliver or if the baby is having trouble and needs to be delivered quickly. In some cases, *forceps* are used to help deliver the baby's head.

- Forceps look like two large salad spoons. They are inserted into the vagina and placed on either side of the baby's head.
- As you push, the doctor gently pulls to help deliver the baby.
- Another method is *vacuum delivery,* also called *vacuum extraction.*
- In this instance, a soft plastic cup is placed on baby's head. Suction is then applied to hold the cup on baby's head.
- As you push, your doctor can gently pull on the suction cup to help deliver your baby.

Removal of the Placenta

Manual Removal

- The placenta is usually expelled with a few contractions following delivery, so manual removal of the placenta is not a procedure that has to be done often.

- When the placenta doesn't come out with contractions (that happen naturally or that can be induced through medication), it may have to be removed by your doctor.
- To do this, he or she places a gloved hand inside the vagina far enough to reach the placenta and assists in delivering it.

D&C for a Retained Placenta

- In some cases, pieces of placenta or membranes can be stuck inside the uterus following delivery. If they cannot be manually removed, a D&C (dilatation & curettage) may need to be done.
- A D&C is done in an operating room. A small tube is placed into the uterus to remove the tissue. This allows the uterus to contract and to stop bleeding.
- You will either have an epidural block for the pain or you will be given general anesthesia.

Tubal Ligation after Delivery?

Some women choose to have a tubal ligation (sterilization) done while they are in the hospital after having their baby. The surgery involves blocking a woman's

Fallopian tubes to prevent further pregnancies. This is an important decision, so take some time to think about it if you are interested.

- Being sterilized following delivery of a baby has some advantages.
- You're in the hospital and won't need another hospitalization.
- If you have an epidural, it's possible to use the epidural as anesthesia for a tubal ligation.
- If you didn't have an epidural, it may be necessary to put you to sleep.
- The procedure may also be done the morning after you've had your baby.
- Having a tubal ligation does not usually lengthen the time you're in the hospital.
- There are also disadvantages to having a sterilization at this time.
- Tubal ligations can be reversed, but it's expensive and requires a hospital stay of 3 to 4 days. Reversals are about 50% effective, but pregnancy cannot be guaranteed. You should consider the procedure permanent and not reversible.
- If you have your tubes tied within a few hours or a day after having your baby, then change your mind, you may regret having the tubal ligation.
- There are several ways to perform tubal ligation.

- The most common is a small incision underneath your bellybutton, through which the Fallopian tubes can then be seen.
- A piece of the tube can be removed, or a ring or clip can be placed on the tube to block it.
- This type of surgery usually requires 30 to 45 minutes to perform.

Tubal Ligation May Be an Option for You

Billy and Lana had always planned on two children, a boy and a girl. Jason would turn 3 in a couple of months and was more of a handful than they had ever imagined. Both Billy and Lana commented, "I'd love to have that kind of energy!"

Now they had been blessed with a daughter. During labor and delivery, Sara, their precious little girl, had swallowed (the doctors and nurses said *aspirated*) meconium. It was explained to the couple that meconium is the first bowel movement or discharge from a baby, made up of mucus and bile. A problem can arise when baby swallows the meconium because it can irritate the lungs and cause a serious pneumonia.

The meconium had been a surprise during Sara's delivery, and the doctors and nurses had reacted quickly to suction it out. Sara had been rushed to the nursery and was receiving oxygen therapy and treatment to help clear her lungs. There was even talk she might have to be transported by helicopter to a higher-level nursery at the university hospital.

(continued on next page)

(continued from previous page)

When the doctor came back in the room to talk to them, she reassured them this was a complication they had to deal with frequently and that babies usually got through it OK, but there was reason for concern. She said it would be several hours before they would know Sara was out of the woods.

Lana had planned on having a tubal ligation after Sara's birth. She had talked to the doctor about it at her first prenatal visit and had signed the necessary papers. There really hadn't been any question for her or Billy about the procedure.

Now the doctor was asking if they wanted to go ahead with the procedure or if they should postpone it. She said again she thought Sara would be fine, but things were a little uncertain right now. She also explained that a tubal ligation should be considered permanent. Some couples decide at a later time to undo or reverse the procedure, but it can be expensive and isn't always successful.

Lana and Billy asked for a few minutes alone to talk about it. When they asked their doctor to come back in, they said they wanted to wait on the surgery. The couple felt it was best to focus on Sara and her condition. They realized the tubal ligation could be done at another time. The doctor agreed with the plan, and they all felt good about the decision.

Glossary

Some Test and Procedure Terms You May Want to Know

Your doctor and his office staff will probably use many medical terms during your pregnancy. You may not have heard some of them before, and this can be very confusing for you. We have included this list of terms related to tests and procedures so you will know what your doctor or nurse is talking about. If you hear a new word and don't know what it means, look it up here.

Abdominal measurement Measurement of the baby's growth in the uterus, taken at prenatal visits. Measurement is from the pubic symphysis to the fundus. Too much growth or too little growth may indicate problems.

Acquired immune deficiency syndrome (AIDS) Debilitating, frequently fatal illness that affects the body's ability to respond to infection. Caused by the human immunodeficiency virus (HIV).

Alpha-fetoprotein (AFP) Substance produced by the unborn baby as it grows inside the uterus. Large amounts of AFP are found in amniotic fluid. Abnormal amounts may reveal neurological problems, such as spina bifida, severe liver or kidney disease, bone problems, blockages or Down syndrome.

Amniocentesis Process by which amniotic fluid is removed from the amniotic sac for testing; fluid is tested for some genetic defects and for fetal lung maturity.

Antibodies Protein substances in the blood produced as a result of a foreign substance being introduced into the blood.

Apgar score Scoring system used to evaluate baby's response to birth, done at 1 and 5 minutes after birth.

Basal body temperature Temperature taken daily to predict ovulation.

Biophysical profile Method of evaluating a fetus in the 3rd trimester before birth. Five areas are evaluated, scored and added together.

Bishop score Method of scoring used to predict the success of inducing labor. Scoring includes dilatation, effacement, station, consistency and position of the cervix. A score is given for each area, then they are added together to give a total score; helps doctor decide whether to induce labor.

Blood pressure Push of blood against the walls of the arteries, which carry blood away from the heart. Changes in blood pressure may indicate problems.

Blood typing Test to determine if a woman's blood type is A, B, AB or O.

Blood-pressure check Measurement of a woman's blood pressure. High blood pressure can be significant during pregnancy, especially nearer the due date. Changes in blood pressure readings can alert the doctor to potential problems.

Carrier Individual who has a recessive disease-causing gene. A carrier usually shows no symptoms but can pass the mutant gene on to his or her children.

Cervical cultures Tests done for infections, including STDs (sexually transmitted diseases); when a Pap smear is done, a sample may also be taken to check for chlamydia, gonorrhea or other STDs.

Chadwick's sign Dark-blue or purple discoloration of the mucosa of the vagina and cervix during pregnancy. Can be seen when a pelvic exam is done.

Chorionic villi Microscopic projections of tissue that make up the placenta.

Chorionic villus sampling (CVS) Diagnostic test that can be done early in pregnancy to determine fetal abnormalities. A biopsy of placental tissue is taken from inside the uterus through the abdomen or the cervix.

Chromosomal abnormality Abnormal number or abnormal makeup of chromosomes.

Chromosomes Structures in a cell's nucleus that contain DNA, which transmits genetic information.

Complete blood count (CBC) Blood test to check iron stores and to check for infections.

Congenital problem Problem present at birth.

Conjoined twins Twins connected at some point on the body or head; they may share vital organs. Previously called *Siamese twins.*

Contraction stress test (CST) Test of baby's response to uterine contractions; to evaluate fetal well-being in the 3rd trimester.

Crown-to-rump length Measurement from the top of the baby's head (crown) to baby's buttocks (rump).

Dilatation Expansion or opening of the cervix.

Dilatation and curettage (D&C) Surgical procedure in which the cervix is stretched open, and the uterine cavity is scraped or suctioned.

Doppler Device that enhances the fetal heartbeat so the doctor and others can hear it.

Down syndrome (mongolism) Chromosomal disorder in which baby has three copies of Chromosome 21 (instead of two); results in mental retardation, distinct physical traits and various other problems.

Due date (EDC; estimated date of confinement) Date baby is expected to be born. Most babies are born near this date, but only 1 of 20 are born on the actual date.

Eclampsia Convulsions and coma in a woman with pre-eclampsia. Not related to epilepsy. Also see *pre-eclampsia.*

Ectopic pregnancy Pregnancy that occurs outside the uterine cavity, most often in the Fallopian tube.

Effacement Thinning and stretching of the cervix during labor.

Electrode Small wire used in fetal monitoring, attached to the fetal scalp.

Electroencephalogram Recording of the electrical activity of the brain.

Embryo In humans, from conception to 10 weeks of pregnancy.

Epidural block Regional anesthesia that numbs the lower half of the body.

Episiotomy Cut or surgical incision from the back of the vagina toward the anus; used to enlarge the vaginal opening for childbirth.

External cephalic version (ECV) Procedure or technique performed at the end of pregnancy to move a breech baby into the head-down (normal) presentation.

Familial Mediterranean fever screening Blood test performed on people of Armenian, Arabic, Turkish and Sephardic Jewish background to identify carriers of a recessive gene. Permits diagnosis in a newborn so treatment can be started.

Fasting blood sugar Blood test to evaluate the amount of sugar in the blood following a period of fasting. Used to diagnose diabetes.

Fetal anomaly Fetal malformation or abnormal development; birth defect.

Fetal fibronectin (fFN) Test done to evaluate premature labor. A sample of cervical-vaginal secretions is taken; if fFN is present after 22 weeks, it indicates increased risk for premature delivery.

Fetal monitor Device used before or during labor to listen to and to record the fetal heartbeat. Monitoring baby inside the uterus can be external (through maternal abdomen) or internal (through maternal vagina).

Fetoscopy Test that lets doctor look through a fetoscope (a fiber-optics scope) to detect subtle abnormalities and problems in a fetus.

Fetus Refers to the unborn baby after 10 weeks of pregnancy until birth.

Fibroids (leiomyoma; myomas) Benign growths or tumors of the uterine muscle.

Follicle-stimulating hormone (FSH) Hormone produced in the pituitary gland that helps an egg in the ovary mature then be released.

Forceps Instrument that fits around the baby's head; used to assist in delivery.

Fundus Top part of the uterus; often measured during pregnancy.

General anesthesia Use of gas and I.V. drugs to produce a sleeplike state for surgery.

Genes Basic units of heredity. Each gene carries specific information and is passed from parent to child. A child receives half of its genes from its mother and half from its father. Every human has about 100,000 genes.

Genetic counseling Consultation between a couple and medical and social-service specialists about genetic defects and/or the possibility of genetic problems in a pregnancy.

Genetic screening tests Various screening and diagnostic tests done to predict whether a couple may have a child with a genetic defect. Usually part of genetic counseling.

Gestational diabetes Occurrence of diabetes during pregnancy (gestation).

Glucose Sugar present in the blood; it is the main source of fuel for the body.

Glucose-tolerance test (GTT) Blood test done to evaluate the body's response to sugar. Blood is drawn from the mother-to-be once or at intervals following ingestion of a sugary substance.

Group-B streptococcal (GBS) infection Infection occurring in the mother's vagina, bladder or rectum. Usually has no symptoms in the mother-to-be, but it can be very serious if the baby contracts it during birth.

Group-B streptococcus (GBS) test Near the end of the pregnancy, samples may be taken from the mother-to-be's vagina, perineum and rectum to check for GBS. A urine test may also be done. If the test is positive, treatment may be started or it may be given during labor.

Hematocrit Proportion of red blood cells to whole blood volume. Important in diagnosing anemia.

Hemoglobin Pigment in red blood cells that carries oxygen to body tissues.

Hepatitis-B antibodies test Test to determine if a person has ever been exposed to hepatitis-B.

Hepatitis-B virus (HBV) Virus that attacks the liver; can cause damage leading to cirrhosis, chronic hepatitis and cancer.

Heritability Degree to which a characteristic is determined by genetics.

HIV test Test to determine if a woman has HIV (the test cannot be done without the woman's knowledge and permission).

Home uterine monitoring Contractions of a pregnant woman's uterus are recorded at home, then transmitted by telephone to the doctor. Used to identify women at risk of premature labor.

Human chorionic gonadotropin (HCG) Hormone produced in early pregnancy; measured in a pregnancy test and a quantitative HCG test.

Human immune-deficiency virus (HIV) Virus that attacks the immune system and causes AIDS.

Hypertension, pregnancy-induced High blood pressure that occurs during pregnancy.

Hyperthyroidism Increased levels of thyroid hormone in the bloodstream.

Hypotension Low blood pressure.

Hypothyroidism Low or inadequate levels of thyroid hormone in the bloodstream.

Hysterosalpingogram (HSG) X-ray performed with contrast dye; dye is injected through the cervix to examine the Fallopian tubes and lining of the uterus.

Hysteroscopy Procedure similar to laparoscopy; a scope is placed through the vagina and cervix to look inside the uterus. It is used to diagnose and to treat fibroids, adhesions or a uterine septum (membrane dividing the uterine cavity). It is performed in an operating room or in the doctor's office, in some cases. A camera is used so pictures can be taken and/or a video can be recorded.

Imaging tests Tests that look inside the body, including X-rays, CT scans (or CAT scans) and magnetic resonance imaging (MRI).

Incompetent cervix Cervix that dilates prematurely and painlessly, without contractions.

Intrauterine-growth restriction (IUGR) Inadequate growth of the fetus during pregnancy.

Isoimmunization Development of specific antibodies directed at the red blood cells of another individual, such as a baby in utero. Occurs when an Rh-negative woman carries an Rh-positive baby or when an Rh-negative woman is given Rh-positive blood.

Karyotype Description of the number and structure of an individual's chromosomes.

Kick count Record of how often a woman feels her baby move; used to evaluate fetal well-being.

Laparoscopy Surgical procedure used to inspect the female organs, including the uterus, tubes and ovaries. It is performed by placing a small telescope (an endoscope) through a ½-inch incision under the bellybutton (umbilicus). A camera is attached to the laparoscope so pelvic organs can be seen on a screen; they can also be recorded on video and pictures can be taken. Used to diagnose endometriosis, adhesions (scar tissue), cysts on the ovaries or abnormalities of the uterus, such as fibroids.

Local anesthesia Use of medications to control pain in specific areas of the body.

Luteinizing hormone (LH) Hormone produced by the pituitary gland that helps an egg in the ovary to mature then be released.

Mammogram X-ray study of the breasts to identify normal and abnormal breast tissue.

Marker Gene or other segment of DNA whose position is known and whose inheritance can be monitored.

McDonald's cerclage (cervical cerclage) Surgical procedure performed for an incompetent cervix. A drawstring-type suture holds the cervical opening closed during pregnancy. See *incompetent cervix.*

Meconium Green or brown substance in the bowels of the fetus; baby's first bowel movement.

Miscarriage Spontaneous loss of pregnancy before 20 weeks.

Multiple-markers tests See *quad-screen test* and *triple-screen test.*

Mutation Change in a gene or chromosome that causes a disorder or causes the inherited susceptibility to a disorder.

Neural-tube defects Abnormal development of the fetal spinal cord and brain, such as spina bifida.

Noninvasive test Any test that doesn't require entering the body or puncturing the skin.

Nonstress test Test in which movements of the baby felt by the mother or observed by a healthcare provider are recorded, along with changes in the fetal heart rate. Used to evaluate fetal well-being.

Nuchal translucency screening Detailed ultrasound that allows the doctor to measure the space behind baby's neck. When combined with blood-test results, can predict a woman's risk of her baby having Down syndrome.

Overdue baby When a baby remains in the uterus beyond 42 weeks.

Ovulation Release of an egg from one of the ovaries.

Oxytocin Drug used to cause contractions and induce labor.

Pap smear Routine screening test that evaluates presence of precancerous or cancerous conditions of the cervix.

Pelvic exam Physical examination by the doctor, who feels inside the vagina to evaluate the size of the uterus at the beginning of pregnancy. Also done toward the end of pregnancy to help determine if the cervix is dilating and thinning.

Percutaneous umbilical blood sampling (PUBS; cordocentesis) Test done on the fetus to diagnose Rh-incompatibility, blood disorders and infections.

Pituitary gland Gland at the base of the brain that controls growth in the body.

Placenta Tissue that provides nourishment to the fetus and takes waste away from the fetus.

Postdate pregnancy Pregnancy that extends beyond 42 weeks.

Pre-eclampsia Combination of serious symptoms unique to pregnancy, including high blood pressure, edema, swelling and changes in reflexes.

Progesterone Female hormone produced in the ovaries that stimulates maturation of the lining of the uterus.

Prostaglandin Chemical made in the body with many effects, including tightening of the uterus.

Pubic symphysis Bony prominence in the pelvic bone found in the middle of a woman's lower abdomen. This bony area is just above your urethra (where urine comes out), 6 to 10 inches below the bellybutton, depending on how tall you are. It may be felt 1 or 2 inches below your pubic hairline. It is the landmark from which the doctor often measures the growing uterus during pregnancy.

Quad-screen test Measurement of four blood components to help identify fetal problems. The four tests include alpha-fetoprotein, human chorionic gonadotropin, unconjugated estriol and inhibin-A.

Recessive inheritance Mutation that must be inherited from *both* parents for baby to be affected. Carrier parents are usually unaffected because each has only one copy of the mutant gene.

Rh-factor Blood test to determine if a woman is Rh-negative.

Rh-negative Absence of rhesus antibody in the blood.

Rh-sensitivity See *isoimmunization.*

RhoGAM Medication given during pregnancy and following delivery to prevent isoimmunization. See *isoimmunization.*

Ripening Softening of the cervix before labor.

Rubella titer Blood test to check for immunity against rubella (German measles).

Sex chromosomes Chromosomes that determine the sex of an individual. Women have two X chromosomes, and men have an X and a Y chromosome.

Sexually transmitted disease (STD) Infection transmitted through sexual contact or sexual intercourse.

Sickle-cell anemia Anemia caused by abnormal red blood cells shaped like a sickle or a cylinder.

Speculum Instrument used to open the vagina so the cervix can be seen.

Sperm count (semen analysis) Microscopic exam of semen.

Spina bifida Birth defect in which membranes of the spinal cord and/or the spinal cord itself protrude outside the protective bony canal of the spine. Can cause paralysis or malfunction of lower extremities.

Spinal block Regional anesthesia that numbs the lower half of the body.

Station Describes amount of descent of the baby into the birth canal.

Stillbirth Loss of a pregnancy any time after 20 weeks.

Stress test See *contraction stress test.*

Syphilis Sexually transmitted disease caused by the organism *Treponema pallidum.*

Syphilis test Test for syphilis; if a woman has syphilis, treatment will be started.

Thrombophilia Disorder of the hemopoietic system (system that controls formation of blood cells) that causes the blood to clot when it shouldn't; this disorder can lead to complications in both mother and baby. Blood clots from thrombophilias can be serious for the fetus because they have been related to miscarriage, stillbirth, early or severe pre-eclampsia, placental abruption and intrauterine-growth restriction.

Trimester Divisions of pregnancy, approximately 13 weeks each.

Triple-screen test Measurement of three blood components to help identify fetal problems. The three tests include alpha-fetoprotein, human chorionic gonadotropin and unconjugated estriol.

Trisomy Presence of an extra copy of a chromosome; there are three copies instead of two. The most common is trisomy 21, which causes Down syndrome.

Ultrasound (sonogram; sonography) Noninvasive test that shows a picture of the fetus inside womb. Sound waves bounce off fetus to create a picture.

Urinalysis and urine cultures Tests for infections and to determine the levels of sugar and protein in the urine.

Vacuum extraction Use of a rubber or plastic cup with suction; applied to baby's head to assist in delivery.

Weight check Weight is checked at every prenatal visit; gaining too much weight or not gaining enough weight can indicate problems.

X chromosome One of the two sex chromosomes; women have two X chromosomes.

X-ray An imaging test that uses electromagnetic radiation to take pictures inside the body.

Y chromosome One of the two sex chromosomes; men have one X chromosome and one Y chromosome. If the man contributes an X chromosome, the baby will be a girl. If he contributes a Y chromosome, the baby will be a boy.

Also by Glade B. Curtis, M.D., M.P.H., OB/GYN and Judith Schuler, M.S.

Your Pregnancy Week by Week, 5th Edition
ISBN: 1-55561-346-2 (paper)
1-55561-347-0 (cloth)

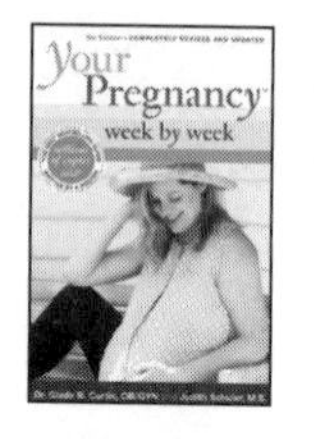

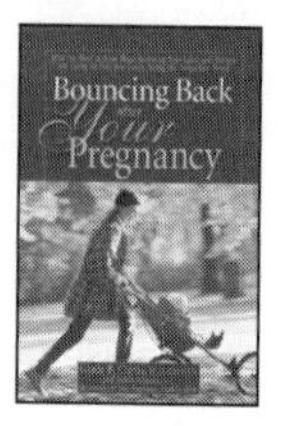

Bouncing Back After Your Pregnancy
ISBN: 0-7382-0606-7

Your Baby's First Year, Week by Week
ISBN: 1-55561-232-6 (paper)
1-55561-257-1 (cloth)

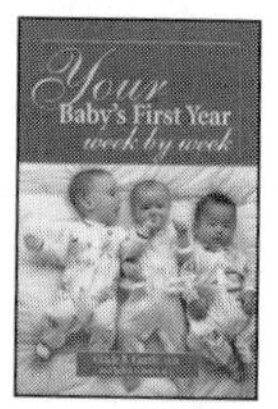

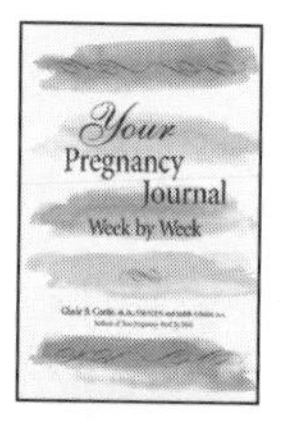

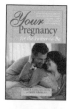

Your Pregnancy Journ
Week by Week
ISBN: 1-55561-343-8

Your Pregnancy for the Father to Be
ISBN: 0-7382-1002-1

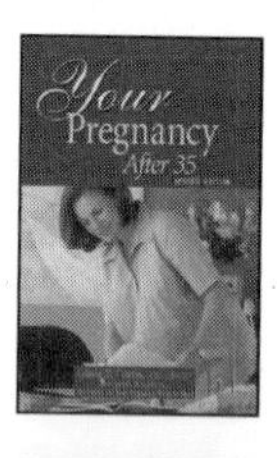

Your Pregnancy After .
ISBN: 1-55561-319-5

Your Pregnancy Questions and Answers
ISBN: 0-7382-1003-X

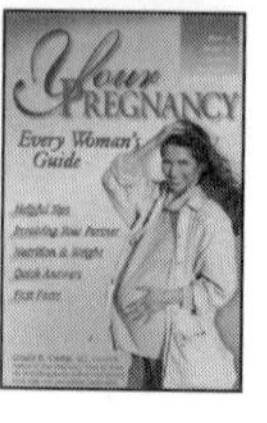

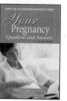

Your Pregnancy: Every Woman's Guide
ISBN: 0-7382-1001-3

Da Capo Lifelong Books are available wherever books are sold and at special discounts for bulk purchases in the U.S. by corporations, institutions, and other organizations. For more information, please contact the Special Markets Department at the Perseus Books Group, 11 Cambridge Center, Cambridge, MA 02142, or call (800) 255-1514, or e-mail special.markets@perseusbooks.com.